THE PRITIKIN
WEIGHT LOSS
BREAKTHROUGH

THE PRITIKIN® WEIGHT LOSS BREAKTHROUGH

FIVE EASY STEPS TO OUTSMART YOUR FAT INSTINCT

ROBERT PRITIKIN

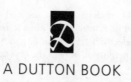

A DUTTON BOOK

A NOTE TO THE READER

Nothing written in this book should be viewed as a substitute for competent medical care. Also, you should not undertake any changes in diet or exercise patterns without first consulting your physician, especially if you are currently being treated for any risk factor related to heart disease, high blood pressure, or adult-onset diabetes.

to my father, Nathan Pritikin

ACKNOWLEDGMENTS

I would like to begin by acknowledging my co-author, Kevin Wiser, without whom I would never have completed this project, and writer Tom Monte, who took our ideas and put them into words. My heartfelt gratitude goes out to both of them.

As I began to explore and refine my early ideas, the scientists, nutritionists, and staff at the Pritikin Longevity Center proved to be essential to my understanding of the fat instinct. The head of nutritional research, Dr. Jay Kenney, identified and simplified the scientific literature linking food choices to satiety, insulin, weight gain, and weight loss. Our director of science, Dr. William McCarthy, introduced me to a series of powerful hypotheses, including J.P. Flatt's concepts on the impact of exercise on food preferences. Working with Pritikin Lifestyle counselors Mary Nakata and Andrea Siegman, Dr. McCarthy also helped shape my understanding of the emotional and behavioral triggers that lead to relapse. I recognized our instinctual craving for fat, but these people helped to give my ideas a scientific foundation. Moreover, their thoughts and analyses helped me understand how people successfully create and adhere to healthy ways of living—or how they outsmart the fat instinct.

The ideas that flowed from all of these people would never have come together as a logical, cohesive picture were it not for Kevin Wiser. Kevin has a gift for breaking down complex information and organizing it into simple, rational concepts that hold up under scientific scrutiny, yet can be understood by anyone. Every new thought I have must pass the "KW" gauntlet for logic, accessibility, and relevance. The developing theory of the fat instinct was no different. In fact, it was Kevin who, after the two of us had already spent innumerable hours wrestling with these concepts, coined the term "the fat instinct." Together, Kevin and I put together a new series of talks that I gave that formed the basis for the theory and this book.

No program for good health works without tasty and practical foods and recipes. Susan Massaron, our cooking school instructor, and Nicolas Klontz, our executive chef, were the artists behind our recipes. Susan, along with our talented dietitians, Diane Grabowski-Nepa and Maria McIntosh, created the meal plans. These plans came out of years of practical experience born of helping people adapt to healthier ways of eating.

Dr. James Barnard was responsible for all of the published clinical results of the Pritikin Program. My father always said that if it weren't for Dr. Barnard, we never would have published anything. It is our published research that forms the foundation and credibility for our program.

Once we had our ideas in place, Tom Monte took our lecture "Outsmarting the Fat Instinct" and turned it into this book. He was the only choice as our writer. My father always said that Tom would write his biography and indeed he did, with my mother, Ilene Pritikin. Tom has the ability to take complicated scientific ideas and turn them into a compelling story. If this book entertains as well as informs, Tom deserves a great deal of the credit.

I want to thank Augieo Nieto, president of Life-Fitness, whose unique motorized treadmill machine helps to keep me fit and has allowed me to resume my passion for running. I also thank our executive secretary April Murphy, whose tireless work and upbeat spirit helps to make the atmosphere at the Pritikin Longevity Center a little more efficient and joyful each day.

This presentation of the fat instinct arose after taking the existing scientific research and synthesizing that information into a new approach to health. But such a synthesis would not have been possible without the contributions made by our incredibly talented staff of professionals representing medicine, nutrition, exercise physiology, behavior science, cooking, and lifestyle engineering. Each of these people has made invaluable contributions to my understanding of health and to this book, and I thank you all.

And finally, it was my mother who reviewed and edited the book. To this day, my mother corrects my English and reorganizes my thinking. Everyone should have such a loving editor.

Contents

I grew up watching my father, Nathan Pritikin, adhere perfectly to a diet and exercise regimen that modern science has described as the healthiest ever created. It was a paradoxical fate. On one hand, I was deeply inspired by my father, a man who single-handedly changed the lives of millions of people, but I was also frustrated by his example. While he seemed to be motivated exclusively by reason and science, I was driven—at least some of the time—by my irrational instincts. While he was eating brown rice, vegetables, fruit, and an occasional piece of fish, I was feeling the urge to eat a hamburger, drown my salad in an oily dressing, and finish my meal with a piece of chocolate cake. While he walked the straight and narrow path, I was wandering in the forest.

None of my behaviors ever seemed to upset him. In the most gentle, objective terms, he would encourage me to eat a lot of small, healthy meals throughout the day, to exercise regularly, and to try to stick to a healthy diet. Then he'd go out and run three miles. What I didn't realize then was that my father was covertly describing a way of life that could overcome my instinctual urges and make me crave foods that would protect my health.

Admittedly, my father had reasons for living by the letter of the law that I didn't have. In the late 1950s, he was diagnosed with "incurable" heart disease, which is what prompted him to create his program in the first place. I was fresh out of the first grade—the year was 1958—when our family began eating a strange diet made up primarily of unprocessed grains, lots of fresh vegetables, fruit, and fish. This was long before there was even a hint of what might be called the modern diet and health revolution. While my friends were eating Swanson TV dinners, my family was dining on brown rice, corn, wheat, and barley;

all kinds of green, yellow, and orange vegetables; beans; homemade vegetable soups; and fruit desserts.

Although the program my father created came to be known as the Pritikin Program, it has a great deal in common with the traditional human diet that much of humanity still subsists on. But in the 1950s, the world was being transformed by new cars, television sets, and appliances, all of which defined your standing as an American. Among the most important status symbols at the time were big fatty steaks and TV dinners, foods my father was saying were bad for your health. Needless to say, everyone I knew thought we were strange and, frankly, so did I.

Strange or not, my father's program cured his heart disease and launched him as the pioneer spokesman for a dietary approach to the illness. As he said at the time, "From that point on, I knew I would try to convert everyone in the world to a new way of living." Over the next thirty years, my father counseled people privately on their health for free; conducted his own research on the use of diet and exercise as a treatment for heart disease, diabetes, and other serious illnesses; and opened the Pritikin Longevity Center, where he and his medical staff used his program to restore health to tens of thousands of people.

My father had additional incentives, as well. For most of his adult life he struggled with a worrisome blood abnormality not understood by his medical doctors, which eventually became a life-threatening cancer. This was further inducement for my father to follow his program to the letter. Yet, he never did anything out of coercion or any sense of fear. On the contrary, he loved his diet and exercise routine. Even more, he loved science and the pursuit of knowledge. My father had a passion for uncovering the secrets of the human body, for burrowing deeply into the mysteries of health and illness.

In 1985 my father died and I took over the Pritikin Longevity Center. In addition to having a background in science, I had been working with my father for ten years at that point, including assisting him on his first big research project, the Long Beach Veteran's Administration Study in which he demonstrated the efficacy of his program for treating heart disease, diabetes, and other serious illnesses.

At the center, over the course of many years, I had the opportunity to meet thousands of people who were struggling with issues related to diet and health. Like my father, I was sympathetic to their dilemma, but for different reasons. A compassionate person by nature, he would spend hours talking to people about any difficulties they had staying on the program, even though he didn't have those problems himself. My father had an eminently simple and rational approach to life that, in certain ways, precluded him from understanding human complexity. He believed, as many scientists do, that if you give people the right information, they will automatically change their behavior. For example, his approach to the problem of cigarette smoking was simply to explain the effects of carbon monoxide, tars, and nicotine on the body. He believed that such information alone would be enough to convince people to quit, even with the addictive qualities of tobacco. He didn't understand that much of human behavior, especially regarding health, food, and exercise, is instinctual and irrational and that appealing to the intellect alone is sometimes not enough to create lasting change.

I was different. I had the good fortune of being healthy and active, but I knew firsthand how difficult it is to maintain a healthy lifestyle in the face of many well-advertised temptations. I could empathize with many of the people who attended the lectures I gave around the country, or read our books, or came to the Longevity Center for whom sticking to a healthful diet was a constant challenge.

My father must have sensed that quality in me. Twenty years ago he told me, "Robert, today we have to worry about getting people on a healthy diet. Ten years from now, we'll have to figure out how to keep them on it." My father worked so hard at getting the message out that he never got around to figuring out how to find a way to help people maintain a healthy way of life, given all the obstacles we all face in the modern world. That job was left to the next generation of Pritikin researchers and to me.

THE PRITIKIN LONGEVITY CENTER

The Pritikin Longevity Center, located in Santa Monica, California, and Miami Beach, Florida, is the single biggest experiment in the use of diet and exercise as a treatment for disease ever created. In the two decades of its existence, more than 65,000 people have come to the center, most of them suffering from atherosclerosis, angina, diabetes, high blood pressure, claudication (pain and cramping in the legs due to poor circulation), various degrees of overweight and obesity. Many have already had heart attacks. Some have been scheduled for bypass surgery and have come to the center hoping to avoid it. The Pritikin Program has been more successful at restoring people to normal function without the use of medication than any other therapy known. No other institution in the world can match our experience and expertise in the use of diet and exercise as a treatment for these serious diseases.

The center is also a primary research facility. As of this writing, in 1996, we have conducted more than seventy scientific studies of people attending our center; that research has been published in *The New England Journal of Medicine, Circulation, The Archives of Internal Medicine, The American Journal of Cardiology, Diabetes Care,* and *Cancer* (the journal of the National Cancer Institute), just to name a handful of the scientific publications that have reported our results. Our research has examined the effects of our program on heart disease, diabetes, high blood pressure, and risk factors for breast and prostate cancer. We regularly participate in scientific studies with other leading research institutions, such as the University of California at Los Angeles (UCLA).

Among the many things I have learned since taking over the center is that, essentially, there are two types of people who adopt the Pritikin Program. The first group of people buy a book or come to the center, learn the program, and have no trouble staying on it for life. Many of these people had believed that they were beyond any hope of recovering their health, ideal weight, or vitality. Then they followed the program, regained their health, and got a second chance at living. Many of them know in their hearts that if they go back to their old ways of living, they'll get sick again. I'll share some of their stories with you in this book. But I would learn much later that their adherence to the program is supported by something even more powerful than their joy at being given a second chance. These people cultivate behaviors that overcome their instinctual desire for fat and calorie-rich foods.

The second group of people who adopt our program do their best to maintain the diet and lifestyle, but are driven by their overpowering urges for fat, sugar, and other unhealthful foods. They may go back to their old ways of eating and living, with predictable results.

At first, I thought the main difference between those who maintained a healthy diet and lifestyle and those who didn't was discipline. What else could it be but that some people simply have more willpower than others? But upon closer examination, I realized that there was more to the problem than a lack of discipline. Right now, 40 percent of women and 20 percent of men are on diets, some of which require incredible amounts of discipline to maintain for even one week! Then there are the vast majority of Americans who are trying to improve their health by eating less fat and more whole grains, fresh vegetables, and fruit. People everywhere are trying to do better. Nevertheless, each year the same old New Year's resolutions are broken, largely because the diets people had hoped would restore their health cannot be followed for very long. The truth is that most people cannot follow a diet, no matter what diet they adopt.

Unfortunately, it shows. The average American gained eight pounds in the last ten years. Overweight and obesity have become epidemic in the West, not only among adults, but increasingly among children. Television commercials advertise products that are purportedly "low in fat" and "high in fiber," but Americans are getting fatter. Heart disease remains the number-one killer of Americans and cancer isn't far behind.

The incongruity between what people want and what people actually do baffled me at first. What is it about fat and, to a lesser extent, sugar that is so difficult to avoid? I kept asking myself. Why do people have such powerful urges for fatty foods? And then I had one of those lightbulb moments, a flash of insight. I formed a hypothesis based upon my observations and then went back to the scientific and medical literature.

For the next three years, my reading of the scientific literature ranged far and wide, from anthropology, archeology, and paleontology, to anatomy, nutrition, and medical science. Working with the research scientists and medical doctors at the Pritikin Longevity Center, I put all the science together into a comprehensive picture, solving a puzzle whose pieces suddenly combined to create a recognizable image. And when we all stood back and looked at that picture, we realized that we had discovered the reason people crave fat and foods rich in calories.

We had uncovered the fat instinct.

DEADLY CRAVING

The foods that are most difficult to give up are those rich in fat and, to a lesser extent, sugar. Not only are they difficult to avoid, but the minute you eat them, you want to eat more, which means they encourage all of us to overeat. Simply put, most people become overweight or develop degenerative diseases because they eat too much fat. Excess fat is by far the most dangerous substance in the food supply and the reason most people become obese or develop degenerative diseases. As my father pointed out more than 30 years ago, excess fat and cholesterol poison the human body—he called the condition "lipotoxemia"—and contribute to a wide array of diseases. The specific illnesses that surface from such poisoning depends on one's genetic vulnerability. One person's genetic weakness may cause him to develop heart disease, while another person becomes obese, someone else gets adult-onset diabetes, and still another is diagnosed with a diet-related cancer.

The solution to the major illnesses caused by lipotoxemia is eating a diet significantly lower in fat and cholesterol, and rich in nutrients and fiber. The problem we face at the Pritikin Longevity Center is helping people to adopt the program and to adhere to it—with minimal effort and maximum satisfaction—for the rest of their lives.

After studying this very problem for years, we have arrived at the solution, which this book will help you accomplish.

Human beings, like many animals, are instinctually driven to eat fat. We have been designed by nature to eat as much fat as we can, whenever the opportunity presents itself. Eating fat is a big part of why the human species survived innumerable famines and still exists today. Fat has the unique characteristic of containing more calories per gram than any other food source; these fat-calories can be stored efficiently on the body and utilized during food shortages and famines that regularly interrupt the food supply. Despite its importance to our survival, fat has been in critically short supply throughout most of human experience. We had to develop an instinctual craving for fat because it insured that we wouldn't pass up any opportunity to consume it. Now, as throughout human existence, we are being driven by that craving. But today it is killing us because of the different nature of the modern diet which makes fat super-abundant.

FINDING AN ANSWER

The Pritikin researchers didn't stop with the recognition of the fat instinct, however. After considerably more study and experimentation, we found that the fat instinct can be outsmarted by a simple set of behaviors. Not only do these behaviors overcome the fat instinct, but they awaken in us a craving for the foods that can restore our health. This discovery explained why certain people are able to remain on the Pritikin Program and incorporate it easily into their lives without any sense of deprivation. For them, such a lifestyle is natural and easy, because they have stumbled upon the very behaviors that overcome the fat instinct and make a healthy diet delicious and much easier to follow.

Inside each of us is an innate desire for good health, abundant energy, beauty, and the fulfillment of our potential as human beings. As long as the fat instinct controls us, it's far more difficult to achieve these goals. Only by adopting behaviors that tame the fat instinct can we be free to live in ways that will lead us to good health, abundant energy, and a fit body.

This book will show you how you can accomplish these goals. As you read it, you will realize that it's unlike any diet-and-health book you have ever read. I want you to understand your cravings for fat and other calorie-rich foods, such as sugar, in a whole new way. You and I are not going to enter into a silent denial of our cravings for fat and calorie-rich foods. On the contrary, I am going to explore those cravings until you fully understand them and know how to escape their grasp.

At the same time, I'm not going to scare you into changing by concentrating exclusively on the dangers of fat, sugar, and other unhealthful foods. Nor will I use fear to get you to discipline yourself so that you stay on the program. Fear can be a good initial motivating force, but we are so good at rationalizing our fears that it often doesn't work in the long run. Ironically, neither does discipline alone. What works is knowing how you can promote what is good and healthy in yourself. In most cases, the only thing that stands between you and good health is the fat instinct, and I'm going to show you how you can outsmart it so that you can be free to be healthy, attractive, and fully alive.

YEARNING TO BE HEALTHY, BUT LOST ON THE WAY

One of the beauties of the human spirit is that hope springs eternal. That wonderful aspect of our nature is also the source of our vulnerability. All of us want to be healthy and fully alive. The trouble is that unlike the fat instinct, which when triggered produces a very distinct and powerful set of behaviors, our instinctual desire for health doesn't give us a clear direction that might lead to the goal. This is made even worse by the fact that there are so many different kinds of health programs today, many offering conflicting approaches to the promised land. Most of us are willing to try anything, at least once, to achieve our goals. Which means that we can go through a lot of programs before we find the one that actually delivers the goods.

One way to cut through the confusion is to begin with a better understanding of health. Modern medicine defines health as the absence of the symptoms of disease, but you and I know that that's not what health is. That's like describing light as the absence of darkness. Health is the sunlight for which we are searching. But in order to understand health and our yearning for it, we must begin by understanding its importance to the survival of our species.

In the course of our long evolutionary development, those individuals who possessed the characteristics of health were more likely to survive long enough to reach sexual maturity and thus propagate the species. Healthy adults were physically stronger; they could endure the elements and thrive under difficult conditions. A healthy adult male had a greater chance of acquiring a mate, or even numerous mates, than one who was weak or ill. Thus, the healthy male or female was far more likely to reproduce and pass on his or her genes. This, too, enhanced survival.

In time, humans instinctively recognized the importance of health and its desirability. We also learned to perceive the characteristics that were "symptoms" of health. We could spot these traits that made an individual desirable to prospective mates. Over time, a health instinct arose that was also central to survival.

The instinctive longing for the characteristics associated with health have been passed down through tens of thousands of generations because the fundamental attributes of health and fitness are ultimately rooted in promoting life, which is to say, ensuring survival.

Of course, the Darwinian reasons for our desire for healthy and fit mates hardly matter when we are overweight, or when we wake up in the morning and don't feel well, or when we suffer from a serious illness. All of us still yearn to be fit and healthy, no matter what the reasons are. And all we have to do is consider for a moment the qualities and characteristics of health to know how much we want them. They include: abundant energy; physical strength; the ability to live comfortably at our optimal weight; the capacity to enjoy good sleep; a strong appetite; and a healthy and fulfilling sex life. People who have such characteristics can consider themselves blessed. We recognize that health is associated with having a clear mind. It's also fundamental to the expression of our unique talents and characteristics. Health increases the likelihood that we can love and be loved. It also enhances our chances of fulfilling our potential and serving our community in some purposeful way. These characteristics—the "symptoms" of health—make us appealing, even beautiful, and thus increase our chances for attracting a mate, having children, achieving success, and enjoying long life.

Remarkably, everyone who adopts the Pritikin Program and maintains it consistently vastly improve their symptoms of health. I have seen the Pritikin Program transform tens of thousands of people who come to our center, or buy one of our books, when it appears that they are so sick that all is lost. The human organism is extremely resilient; given the right conditions, it can restore health, even when it seems that recovery is beyond reach.

The challenge facing all of us today is this: How do we adopt a healing diet and lifestyle without feeling deprived or constrained by a daily struggle against the temptations of the fat instinct? Frankly, I don't want to have to think too much about what I can and cannot eat, and I cannot live with a program that depends exclusively on discipline. On the other hand, I don't want to be overweight and sick, a slave of my fat instinct. I want to be healthy, not miserable. Therefore, what I really want to know is this: How can I outsmart my fat instinct and, at the same time, promote my health, without having to suffer with a program that feels nearly as uncomfortable as the disease itself? I want to enjoy the foods that make me feel good and look good.

This book is going to show you how to do just that.

Actually, the program that controls the fat instinct and makes us desire the foods that promote health, beauty, vitality, and long life was right under our noses all the time. We just didn't see it because we didn't understand the fat instinct and its power to influence our health and dietary decisions.

If we define health according to the characteristics I outlined above, we have a compass to guide us. We can find people who fit that description, study their diets and behaviors, and shape a program that mimics their way of life. We can try to understand how these people have escaped the power of the fat instinct. And that's exactly what we did at the Pritikin Longevity Center.

We have four groups of people to draw our information from. The first is our own early ancestors, whose diets and behaviors shaped our anatomy and biochemistry. We cannot deny our own anatomy and biochemistry just because the last fifty years have been a lot different from the previous two million.

The second group is composed of populations of people from around the world who avoid obesity and the diseases of affluence. We have studied their diets and lifestyles closely to discover what they are doing that supports their health, and why they haven't been undermined by the fat instinct.

The third group we can look at is comprised of people who have successfully lost weight and then managed to keep that weight off. How did they do it? we wonder. In fact, scientists recently asked that question to nearly 800 men and women who had lost an average of 66 pounds, and then managed to keep that weight off for at least five years. Remarkably, most of the people studied had been obese since childhood and about half had at least one parent who had been obese. The researchers, who in 1997 published their findings in *The American Journal of Clinical Nutrition*, discovered that it was not a high-protein diet, or some recently touted fad nutrient, that was responsible for the weight loss and weight maintenance, but a low-fat diet and exercise program that replicated the Pritikin approach. In fact, these people who had lost enormous amounts of weight, and then kept that weight off, had adopted the very behaviors we recommend—behaviors that outsmart the fat instinct and cause people to lose weight naturally.

The fourth group is the large population of Pritikin alumni, people who have reversed serious diseases—many of them life-threatening—on our program. We have paid particular attention to those people who have little trouble remaining on the program, who, in short, have overcome their fat instinct.

A close examination of these groups reveals that they have certain behaviors in common, and that these behaviors are highly correlated with health, longevity, optimal weight, and adherence to healthy eating. Moreover, these behaviors affect biology and food preferences, and thus help people maintain a healthy way of life.

Finally, we can examine the abundant scientific evidence that points consistently to a diet and lifestyle that promote maximum health, optimal weight, and longevity.

A lot of the time, scientific evidence can seem abstract and far away. But when you apply the understanding to your situation, the information can transform your life, as it did for Betty Winters.

BETTY'S RECOVERY

In 1990, Betty Winters's life started to fall apart. Her husband, who had suffered from tuberculosis for many years, suddenly took a turn for the worse and lost the use of his legs. Once her husband's condition worsened, Betty's nursing assistant decided the job was too hard for her and left. Shortly thereafter, Betty's mother died. Betty was in her late forties, but she could see her own mortality coming on quickly.

These events precipitated a four-year depression during which Betty labored to help her husband during the day and ate chocolate and drank vodka at night. As her mood fell, her blood pressure and blood cholesterol level skyrocketed. So did her weight. She put on fifty pounds. And then in late 1993, she got pneumonia and was hospitalized. When Betty recovered, her doctor told her that her cholesterol level was 266 mg/dl, which is dangerously high. People with cholesterol levels in Betty's range have four times the rate of heart attacks of those with cholesterol levels below 200.

Betty's doctor gave her two choices: either take Mevacor, a cholesterol-lowering drug, or lose weight. Already on high blood pressure medication and hating it, Betty refused the drug and decided to explore other possible treatments. That's when she found a book on the Pritikin Program and used it to transform her life. She gave up meat and oil, and started eating lots of vegetables. "It was fun," Betty recalled. "I love vegetables and I love to cook."

She started to lose weight immediately. She also realized that her spirit was being restored. Betty decided that she was feeling so good from the program that she had to know more, so she spent two weeks at the Miami Pritikin Center, where she fine-tuned her diet and exercise program. When she completed her two-week stay at the Miami Center in April 1994, she was committed to turning her life around.

By April 1995, Betty had lost all fifty pounds and had kept them off. She also had transformed her health, dropping her blood cholesterol from 266 mg/dl to 163 mg/dl. Her triglycerides were 74 (35 to 135 mg/dl is the healthy range). She is off blood pressure medication and she walks every day on her treadmill. "It's the best thing that ever happened to me," she says of her program routine. She feels no sense of deprivation on the diet and is able to maintain it even when she eats out and travels. Consequently, she's more fit and healthy, which has transformed her outlook and the circumstances of her life.

"I hated to think of myself as a victim," Betty told us recently. "But I was. I was caught up in a victim environment, a woe-is-me attitude. I had to give it up, surrender all my destructive feelings, my destructive habits, and move on. My life was at stake. With Pritikin, I've found the strength, the health, to carry me through even the worst days. I've gone from victim to victor! Today I'm healthy and happy," said Betty. "Every morning I wake up feeling good."

Betty is only one of tens of thousands who have transformed their lives on our program. Success begins by understanding the nature of your fat instinct and how to outsmart it. At that point, you can make wise choices without the constant pressure of hunger, feelings of deprivation, and the constant craving for high-fat and calorie-rich foods. As your health and vitality improve, as your weight falls and your body becomes fit and trim, you will realize that you have the freedom and the personal power to enjoy your life.

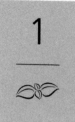

THE FAT INSTINCT
REVEALED

Susan, a thirty-eight-year-old mother of two, is married, has a successful career as a graphic designer, and has gained twenty extra
pounds that she can't get rid of. During her college years, Susan maintained her ideal weight effortlessly. Jealous friends used to joke that
she could "eat anything" and remain a perfect size 9. But her first
pregnancy changed all that; Susan ballooned and stayed that way,
even after she gave birth. Susan promised herself that she would
regain her figure and youthful vitality. She didn't realize how tough it
would be to keep that promise.

Right away, she adopted a diet, counted calories like they were precious stones, routinely deprived herself of foods that she really wanted
to eat, and controlled the portions of those she did eat. She read
books on dieting, health, and discipline.

At first, she reveled in the orderliness and discipline that her new
diet imposed upon her life. And given that her actions were directed
toward a much desired goal—namely, the loss of twenty pounds—the
whole enterprise of dieting inspired her and raised her self-esteem.
Even better were the times she got on the scale and realized she was
losing weight. That was real satisfaction. "You really feel good when
you start a diet and you start losing weight because you see yourself
accomplishing what you set out to do, and you're excited to get your
old body back," she said.

As every experienced dieter knows, the first five to ten pounds are
the easiest to lose, in part because much of it is water. It's the last ten
or twenty pounds that test the spirit and make a person question
whether or not she actually wants to diet. That's what happened to
Susan.

"Eventually, weight loss depends on your willingness to feel bad all the time," Susan said. Pretty soon, the constant pull of hunger, irritability, and cold extremities became intolerable. Her energy levels fluctuated wildly; so did her moods. The whole endeavor of losing weight preoccupied her mind—not because she was more attached to food than anyone else, but because the effort involved so much discomfort. Visions of greasy cheeseburgers, pastries, and whole chocolate cakes danced constantly in her head (that is, when she wasn't experiencing headaches associated with hunger).

Susan realized that she couldn't endure the discomfort of dieting forever, and at some point her discipline just snapped. Before she could rationally get hold of herself, she was eating everything in sight and, in the process, regaining the ten pounds she had lost. Even worse, she realized that when she regained the weight, she lost muscle tone. Despite the fact that she was only in her late thirties, there was the hint in her arms that her flesh had begun to stretch and sag. She knew the extra weight increased her risk of contracting heart disease, diabetes, high blood pressure, and breast and ovarian cancers. But far more immediate was the fact that she couldn't bear the sight of herself and the feeling of carrying around all those extra pounds. That scared Susan. Feelings of disappointment and failure engulfed her. "What is wrong with me?" she kept asking herself.

Susan never stopped believing that she could regain her slender figure, even though she bought new clothing designed to hide the weight. Still, she held on to some of the old clothes, too, the size 9s that she really liked. They were a symbol of who she had been and who she would be again. "I'll be back," she told those clothes, mimicking the Terminator.

One of the darker aspects of weight gain, Susan realized, was that it had affected the intimacy she had formerly enjoyed with her husband. He hadn't criticized her weight, but she knew—if only intuitively—that he was showing less enthusiasm for her because of the way she looked. Susan questioned why she couldn't get to a stable, attractive weight and maintain it as part of a healthy lifestyle? Why does weight loss have to be such an excruciating and elaborate process? Something inside of Susan kept telling her that she should be able to get old and, at the same time, maintain a good figure and mature beauty. Why do

I have to get fat as I age? Lots of people age gracefully, she thought. Why shouldn't I be one of them?

With all of these overt and subtle incentives running through her mind, Susan committed herself once again to losing the weight and found another diet program. As before, she plunged into the hunger pangs of calorie deprivation, the cold extremities, irritability, and energy fluctuations. Once again, she lost ten pounds. And just when she was within a few pounds of her goal, just when fitting into those size 9s was finally within sight, her willpower buckled. Discipline is like a dam that eventually springs a little leak, she realized. When the leak appears, the whole dam collapses at once. "Food, glorious food!" The words from *Oliver!* sang out in Susan's mind. Pretty soon the ten pounds were back, with five of their friends.

One day she got out of bed, looked in the mirror, and realized that she was overweight and starved. Anger flared inside of her. "You're fat. Get used to it," she told her image in the mirror.

Then she got pregnant again. She gave herself license to eat what she wanted during her pregnancy, rationalizing that she would find an effective weight loss program after she gave birth. During those nine months, Susan gained more weight, winding up thirty-five pounds overweight, which was ten pounds more than her doctor recommended she gain during pregnancy.

Naturally, she was elated when she gave birth. But one morning shortly after going home from the hospital, she got out of bed, stood before her mirror, and was suddenly engulfed with a wave of shock and despondency: There in the mirror was the image of her mother, overweight, exhausted, and very much beyond her prime. She had become the very woman she had promised herself in college she would never be.

Frank is a forty-five-year-old accountant with a wife and three children. As a former high school basketball player and all-around athlete, Frank has an old ballplayer's aversion to exercise. He likes to eat, though. He's thirty-five pounds overweight, but how he got that way is a mystery to Frank. As a high school athlete, Frank never gave any thought to how he would maintain his 6'-2", 170-pound build. In high school and college, he was active without even thinking about it.

Exercise? He had so much fun playing ball that the word never even occurred to him. Of course, times change. He got a job in his profession, got married, had children, and hit forty. From that moment, the physical changes occurred with the inexorable oncoming of night. One day, he played a pickup basketball game with his son and was heaving for air before either one of them had 5 points. "I guess my days of hoop are over," he told himself, without giving it a second thought. For a couple of years, he resisted the fact that he was gaining weight, especially in his stomach. Instead, he continued to wear the same waist-size that he wore in college by lowering his belt further down on his waist. Soon, his pants were four inches lower on his abdomen and he no longer could see his belt buckle. What really hurt, though, was when his wife started dropping subtle—and not so subtle—hints that he was gaining weight and had to start dieting. She said things in restaurants like, "Honey, do you think you should order that steak?" or "I think you're a little *big* for dessert, don't you, honey."

Gradually, Frank was forced to accept that he was no longer a jock. And then one night, as he prepared for bed, he looked into the mirror and realized that he had a belly that was out of control, a double chin, and jowls. "I've got to lose weight," he realized. The thought was sad and a little frightening. "I never had to think about my weight," he said. "And I never thought I'd have to. I guess I never thought I would get old."

The problem was that Frank didn't feel old. Something inside of him kept saying that at forty-five or even fifty-five, he shouldn't look old, either. "There are guys who don't look old when they're sixty-five," Frank said later on. "Why should I look old at forty-five? I feel young inside. I should be thin, you know, light, and have lots of energy. You get to be forty-five, you start succeeding at your work, and you want to enjoy life. You don't want to be old and fat."

Frank was never one for structured diet programs. He figured he could lose the weight simply by exercising and denying himself meals. He started skipping breakfast and, instead, went to the health club. At the club, he walked on the treadmill, pumped some iron, and did the Stairmaster. At noon, he had a light lunch—usually cottage cheese and a diet Coke—and then struggled through the afternoon, suffering from hunger, fatigue, and increasing irritability. When he got home at 6 P.M., Frank was ravenous and grouchy. Then he faced his toughest test. Could he eat a light dinner and then push himself away from the table before his discipline gave way and he gorged on everything but the plates? Remarkably, he managed to do just that on more nights than he cares to remember. Every time he accomplished this remarkable feat of discipline, however, he was rewarded with an evening of pure misery. Frank winces when he recalls making those frequent trips to the kitchen, opening and closing cabinet doors, hoping to find a light snack but confronting only temptation. On such nights, he drank water and ate celery sticks, but such rations had the paradoxical effect of making him even more aware of his hunger. He went to bed with the small reward of knowing he'd done the right thing, or so he thought. But that wasn't good enough. The next day, he skipped breakfast, exercised at the gym, and went to lunch at noon feeling mildly depressed. At the restaurant, he decided to avoid carbohydrates because he had read that they increase weight. Better order a high-protein meal, he told himself. The article said that high protein caused weight loss. Frank ordered a hamburger and a diet Coke. He was still hungry when he went back to work.

At dinner that night, his desire to eat was fortified by the memory of last night's fast. "Not another one like that," he promised himself. This time, his hunger was overwhelming, especially his craving for fatty and salty foods, such as pizza, chips, and salted nuts. Frank decided that he was going to make up for the previous night by giving himself just what he was craving. Before he realized it, however, he was eating seconds and even thirds. "I'll lose the weight tomorrow," he told himself later, only half believing it. The following day, he fasted at breakfast and lunch again, and gorged at dinner. This became his daily pattern.

Frank rationalizes his big dinner meals with the fact that he doesn't eat all day long—that's got to count for something! But the mirror and the bathroom scale disabuse him of this illusion. He's gaining weight! "How do you figure that?" he asks, incredulously. "I'm fasting most of the day and I'm getting fatter!"

Frank and Susan are no different from tens of millions of other dieters: They are victims of the fat instinct, one of the most powerful aspects of our will to survive. In order to fully understand the fat instinct and its enormous power over us, we have to understand how it arose in the first place.

IN THE FOREST: FEAST OR FAMINE

Let me take you back through the long tunnel of time to a point in human evolution when the modern humans, the first Adam and Eve, were born into the original garden, namely the African forest. Modern humans appeared more than two hundred thousand years ago, but we weren't much different from our earlier ancestors, *Homo habilis* (the so-called toolmaker, who lived about two million years ago) and *Homo erectus* (who had much bigger brains than *H. habilis* and lived about five hundred thousand years ago). In fact, anatomists, anthropologists and paleontologists will tell you that the human anatomy—especially our digestive tract—probably has undergone very little change in the last two million years. The big changes have occurred primarily in the nervous system, especially in the size of the brain.

Throughout our entire evolution, our ancestors faced an array of terrible threats to their survival, but perhaps the greatest of these was their unpredictable food supply. Anthropologists tell us that humans didn't start cultivating food until about ten thousand years ago, which means that for millions of years our ancestors depended upon nature's wild and capricious bounty to provide them with what they needed to survive each day. I say capricious because the food supply was unpredictable and famine was a constant threat.

If you were alive then, you'd probably be thinking some version of the following: "Today, there are wild tubers, some of these leafy things, and fruits to eat. What about tomorrow? Maybe I'll find some more roots or I'll find a fallen animal. Or maybe there will be no food at all. I better eat all that I can of what nature provides me today because tomorrow I may starve."

For most of the year, our ancestors ate the foods that were most available, which were starchy roots, tubers, vegetables, and fruit. These plant foods are high in fiber and bulk, but low in calories. They met their immediate caloric needs—meaning they provided enough energy to get them through today and part of tomorrow perhaps, but not much more. This meant that our forebears had to keep eating throughout the day to stay alive. Occasionally, they got lucky. An animal was killed, either by a human hunter or an accident of nature, and those who ate that animal consumed as much of the fat and flesh as they could.

Early humans expended a lot of energy every time they went in search of food, often walking or running for miles in order to find food. Harvesting the food by digging it up or getting it out of trees required additional effort and energy. On top of that, they very often had to flee from predatory animals that wanted to turn Adam and Eve into lunch. It was no picnic out there. The search for food was both exhausting and dangerous. In order to meet their high energy needs, lots of food had to be eaten each day.

Because plant foods provide only enough energy for the short term, they don't give much protection against food shortages, famine, and starvation, the greatest danger early humans faced. During any given scavenging expedition, early humans might find little or nothing to eat; sometimes weeks would pass before they came across a real bounty. As nutritionist Kerin O'Dea, Ph.D., states in the article "Obesity and Diabetes in the 'Land of Milk and Honey,' " published in *Diabetes/Metabolism Reviews*, the Paleolithic diet was characterized by "feast or famine." In order to avoid starvation, our ancestors had to find a food that provided more than enough calories to satisfy not only today's energy needs, but tomorrow's, the day after tomorrow's, and so on. There was only one kind of food that could do that—and that was fat.

A gram of carbohydrate provides 4 calories; a gram of fat provides 9 calories. Clearly, when it comes to surviving famine, fat is the food of choice. As we all know, humans—like other animals—have the ability to store fat in the tissues, which makes it a perfect calorie savings account to be drawn upon when the food supply runs low.

The only problem with fat, at least for our ancestors, was that there wasn't enough of it, partly because they lacked the means to be truly effective hunters. *Homo habilis* may have been called the toolmaker, but he was no Black and Decker man. As archeologists and geologists have discovered, the best tools *H. habilis* had available to him were some crude hand axes, which were essentially stones with chipped edges. Toolmaking gradually increased in sophistication over hundreds of thousands of years, but it wasn't until much later that true knives came into being, which means that our early ancestors were not the most successful big game hunters. Much of their meat consumption came via the generosity of nature: occasionally, an animal that had been killed by another animal or had died by some other means would be found and eaten. That was a happy day.

Still, even when such a feast had been discovered, or killed by a tribesman, there wasn't a lot of fat to go around. Wild animals are lean, especially plant-eating animals, or herbivores. As S. Boyd Eaton, M.D., and Melvin Konner, Ph.D. point out in their study, "Paleolithic Nutrition," published in *The New England Journal of Medicine*: "the nutritional quality of such meat [eaten by early humans] differs considerably from that of meat available in the modern American supermarket; the latter has much more fat. . . . Domesticated animals have always been fatter than their wild ancestors because of their steady food supply and reduced physical activity, but breeding and feeding practices have further increased the proportion of fat to satisfy our desire for tender meat."

Indeed, a modern piece of hamburger meat derives more than 50 percent of its calories from fat. Commonly consumed cuts of beef derive between 40 and 80 percent of their calories from fat. The difference in fat content between a modern domesticated animal and its wild counterpart is often startling. Konner and Eaton note that, "a survey of 15 different species of free-living African herbivores revealed a mean carcass fat content of only 3.9 percent," which is approximately 20 to 25 percent total calories in fat. Even when our early ancestors did eat a piece of meat, the amount of fat they derived from that meat was small in comparison to what we get from meat today. Other animal foods, such as eggs, milk and milk products, and processed meats, like bacon and hot dogs, derive between 50 and 90 percent of their calories from fat.

Little wonder, therefore, that whenever an early human feasted upon a dead animal he immediately gorged on every bit of fat he could extract from the beast. If there was a band of early humans searching the forest for food, and the animal was big enough, the whole scavenging party would sit down and gorge on as much fat and flesh as they could devour. In the fall, seeds and nuts were available throughout the forest, providing early humans with a plant-based source of fat. As with animal fat, people ate as many plant fats as they could.

People didn't gorge because their manners were as primitive as their tools; they gorged out of necessity. In fact, gorging on fat became essential to survival. Our ancestors had to get as much fat into their systems as they could because there was no telling when they would have another feast. Also, if they didn't consume every edible bit of that animal, there was a long line of predators waiting to lay claim to it. Finally, the flesh would rot if left alone, which meant that the feast would be wasted. There was a real time-urgency associated with consumption of animal flesh, and gorging was the only way to respond to it.

Thus, gorging on fat—with its abundance of calories—became a key to survival. But there wasn't a great deal of fat available, especially in the first million years or so of human development when our tool-making skills made us better scavengers than hunters. This made fat a very valuable commodity—indeed, one that was prized and sought after.

When something is essential to the survival of a species, but is in relatively short supply, natural selection may cause that species to adapt its instinctual nature and physical characteristics so that the species can obtain adequate quantities of the needed substance. This is where evolution and natural selection come into the picture, and how humans developed a genetically driven set of behaviors that we have called the fat instinct.

SURVIVAL OF THE FATTEST

Certain characteristics and instincts increase a species' chances of survival because they help it meet the demands of the environment.

Members of the species who have the favorable characteristics and instincts are more likely to survive long enough to procreate, and thereby pass on their genes to their offspring, who will, in turn, also have the same characteristics that enhance survival. Those who do not have these instincts and characteristics often die prematurely, and therefore either do not reproduce, or have fewer offspring. Over a long period of time, the members of the species who have the favorable characteristics will grow in number, while the members with the unfavorable characteristics will gradually die off. In time, the species will be composed exclusively of members who have the beneficial genetic characteristics.

Zoologist and author David Attenborough gives a wonderful example of how such environmental demands determine which characteristics within a given species survive and which ones become extinct. "All individuals of the same species are not identical," writes Attenborough in his book *Life on Earth* (Little, Brown and Co., 1979). "In one clutch of eggs from, for example, a giant tortoise, there will be some hatchlings which, because of their genetic constitution, will develop longer necks than others. In times of drought they will be able to reach [and eat] leaves and so survive. Their brothers and sisters, with shorter necks, will starve and die. So those best fitted to their surroundings will be selected and be able to transmit their characteristics to their offspring. After a great number of generations, tortoises on the arid islands will have longer necks than those on the watered islands."

Our instinct for fat consumption developed in much the same way as the longer necks of tortoises came into being. Our food supply was unpredictable and marked by periodic famine. At some distant point in human existence, a certain number of people were born with a genetic and instinctual preference for fat-rich foods, an instinct that also drove them to gorge on fat whenever they had the chance. This instinctual behavior favored survival, which meant that those who were blessed with this trait were more likely to live long enough to procreate and pass on their genes to their children. The children of these people engaged in the same behavior, survived, and procreated, which meant that over time the fat instinct spread to more and more people. Meanwhile, there were other members of the human race who did not have a strong instinct to overeat high-calorie foods when they had the chance. When food became scarce, these people didn't have the same quantity of calories stored in their tissues—they were too lean—and therefore were more likely to die from starvation during drought and cold winters. Since famine occurred regularly throughout an individual's life, many of those without a strong fat instinct probably died young—too young to have reached sexual maturity and thus have the opportunity to pass on their genes. Over a long period of time, those with the stronger fat instinct survived, while those without it died out. Eventually, the fat instinct grew to be so strong in many populations that it became a fundamental part of our will to survive.

The fat instinct was especially important to the survival of migratory peoples. Polynesians who traveled to distant islands, such as Hawaii, or to the American continents, have a very strong fat instinct. It is easy to understand how people who started long sea voyages to unknown lands were more likely to get there if they had more body fat when they set sail. Only those who had the most calories stored in their tissues—the relatively fat ones—would have survived the longer droughts and colder winters.

Charles Darwin stated that evolution assured survival of the fittest. But a more descriptive way of saying the same thing, at least insofar as humans were concerned, was that survival went to the *fattest*.

THE COUCH POTATO IN ALL OF US

The truth is that given the enormous amount of energy expended just to find food—indeed, just to get through the average day—and the limited amounts of fat available, most of our ancestors would probably be considered fairly slender by modern standards. They had to protect the fat supplies that they carried around on their bodies, which meant that they had to avoid unnecessary work or exercise.

But let's say that as a Paleolithic man or woman, you got the wild idea one day to start jogging through the savanna because you felt like getting some exercise. Well, if a lion or a tiger didn't turn you into breakfast, you'd probably burn off enough calories so that you'd be very hungry when you got home. But on that particular day, perhaps there wasn't much food available at the campsite so you had to go out and look for it. Unfortunately, that was the day a famine started. Guess what? You probably wouldn't get too many more chances to take a little run across the countryside, because the odds are very good that you'd starve to death.

The concept of exercise is ludicrous in an environment in which the fat content of the diet is low and the amount of effort needed to obtain one's food is extremely high. Actually, it's suicidal, because the calories a person expends exercising in such an environment may be the very calories he needs to survive the next famine. We have learned through millions of years of development that burning energy in any needless endeavor—particularly one that is not associated with obtaining food—is not only stupid but dangerous. When Australian aborigines—many of whom still live the Paleolithic way of life—see modern Australians jogging, they crack up with laughter. They think modern people are nuts. Why run after nothing when you have to expend enormous amounts of energy walking or running to find food? It's entirely inconsistent with survival, at least as the aborigines see things.

Conserving calories is not an intellectual decision, any more than craving fat is. It is an instinctual behavior. Nature has programmed us, particularly as adults, to spend as much time as possible lying around, just as adult lions and tigers do in the wild. In other words, the couch potato is in our genes.

THE BODY RESISTS LOSING WEIGHT

There's one more characteristic of the fat instinct that is worth mentioning. After experiencing literally millions of years of food scarcity, your body has been designed to conserve energy during famine. It slows down your metabolic rate every time your calorie consumption drops. Your metabolic rate determines how fast calories are burned as energy. If your metabolic rate is fast, you burn calories rapidly. Demanding exercise, hard work, and stressful events increase your metabolic rate, so that more calories are burned than when you are at rest.

In order to survive famine, all animals, including humans, have developed the physiological ability to respond to a drop in calorie consumption and by slowing down their metabolic rate to conserve calories. This physiological characteristic plays a pivotal role in our modern attempts to lose weight. When you start dieting, your body recognizes the drop in calorie consumption and immediately starts slowing your metabolic rate so that you can survive what your body thinks is a famine. Unfortunately, the slowing of your metabolic rate causes a reduction in the rate at which you burn calories, which means that while you suffer from food deprivation and all the associated discomforts, your body is conserving the fat and calories that you've been trying to burn. That is one of the reasons why those last ten or twenty pounds are so difficult to lose.

THE FOUR CHARACTERISTICS OF THE FAT INSTINCT

The fat instinct is composed of three instinctual behaviors, and one powerful physiological response.

- First, the fat instinct compels us to eat high-fat and calorie-rich foods;

- Second, it drives us, whenever we are hungry, to overeat and, if we are sufficiently hungry, to gorge on rich foods, if they are available;

- Third, it drives us to conserve calories by encouraging us to lie around and avoid any unnecessary expenditures of energy.

- Finally, the fat instinct causes a physiological change in which the body's metabolic rate is dramatically slowed, allowing essential physical activities to continue functioning on fewer calories. Calories are conserved, which means that weight loss is slowed or even stopped entirely.

The fat instinct is always present within you, though much of the time it lies unnoticed until it is triggered by numerous stimuli, including hunger and the sight and smell of fatty or rich foods. Once the fat instinct is triggered, it makes its presence felt through a variety of symptoms that become more intense as you continue to go without adequate calories.

When you miss a meal, or spend a day or two eating slightly less than you're accustomed to eating, you experience hunger pangs and an increased desire for fat and calorie-rich foods. You find hamburgers, steaks, cheese, French fries, and potato chips even more irresistible. Or you could find yourself craving other forms of calorie-rich foods, such as pastries, cakes, croissants, ice cream, or chocolate—foods that are concentrated with calories because of the presence of both fat and sugar. This is the mildest phase of the fat instinct, a phase that most people are satisfying daily.

If you continue to go without adequate calories, and lose more than a few pounds—either because you do not have enough food or because you're dieting—you experience an array of more intense physical discomforts, including: stronger hunger pangs, headache, fatigue, weakness, shaky limbs, anxiety, and a powerful craving for fat and calorie-rich foods. Every dieter is well-acquainted with these symptoms, because they are the very discomforts that defeat dieters every day.

The final phase of the fat instinct, commonly referred to by nutritionists and physicians as the "famine response," is far more significant and severe because it changes the way your body functions and slows or defeats your efforts to lose weight and keep it off. This phase occurs when the body slows its metabolism to conserve its calorie-savings account.

HIGH-FAT FOODS: "BET YOU CAN'T EAT JUST ONE"

One of the aspects of the fat instinct that is so perplexing—and so threatening to human health—is that it compels us to overeat fatty foods. One of the more insidious ways your fat instinct gets you to overeat fat is by dulling your ability to experience fullness, or satiety. This enables you to gorge on great quantities of fat before you feel full.

Of course, all food will fill you up—if you eat enough of it. But different foods give us very different experiences of satiety. Let's say you eat 280 calories of broccoli, and the following day you eat 280 calories of hamburger. Which one will fill you up more? Actually, it's no contest. You probably couldn't eat 280 calories worth of broccoli because you'd have to eat more than two pounds of the stuff. If you eat two pounds of broccoli—assuming you could even get it down—you'd be full for many hours. Yet, you would have eaten only 280 calories.

On the other hand, if you want to eat 280 calories of ground beef, all you have to do is eat 3½ ounces of hamburger meat, which amounts to about the size of a deck of cards—and that's without the bun, cheese, lettuce, tomato, and ketchup! If you add a slice of Monterey Jack cheese to that hamburger, you've added about 125 calories. Put it on a couple of slices of white bread and you've added another 140 calories. But if you want to keep that cheeseburger at around 280 calories, you're going to have to chop the thing in half. Okay, so let's cut the hamburger in half, cut the cheese in half, and use one piece of bread. Now you've got half a cheeseburger that's just about 280 calories. Do you think that's going to fill you up, especially if you're hungry. Not a chance.

The comparison between your average cheeseburger and your average plant food, in this case broccoli, looks like this:

■ 280 calories of broccoli = 2 pounds (plus) or ten cups of broccoli
   Likelihood of experiencing fullness: Certain.

versus

■ 280 calories of cheeseburger = 1.75 ounces of ground beef + 1.75 ounces of Monterey Jack cheese + 1 slice of bread
   Likelihood of experiencing fullness: Small to None.

Fatty foods encourage you to eat more of them because they do not fill you up. But when you eat enough of them to give you the experience of fullness, you also will have eaten a lot more calories than your body needs to function optimally.

A study done by Dr. Susanne Holt and her colleagues at the

Human Nutrition Department at the University of Sydney demonstrated this by measuring the capacity of foods to provide fullness, or satiety. Holt found that when people eat foods rich in fat, or sugar, they are not as satisfied, or full, as they are when they eat the same number of calories from plant foods. Furthermore, these same people were hungrier and ate more food two hours after the high-fat or high-sugar meal than they did two hours after eating fiber-rich, unprocessed plant food.

Holt examined the effects of thirty-eight different foods on forty-one participants, asking each participant to eat specific amounts of a test food (about 250 calories of each food), and then determined how effectively that food filled up the person, or created a feeling of fullness or satiety. Each participant ate an individual test food in the morning, after a 10-hour fast the night before. The participants were given 250 calories of a specific food, along with a glass of water, and then prevented from eating for the next two hours. Over that two-hour period, they were asked to fill out a questionnaire to determine whether or not the food filled them up, and if they still felt hungry. At that point, each participant was allowed to eat freely from a wide variety of foods that were made available to them.

Holt and her colleagues divided the 38 test foods into six categories:

- Fruits, which included grapes, bananas, apples, oranges
- Carbohydrate-rich foods: white bread, whole-meal bread, rye grain bread, white rice, brown rice, white pasta, brown pasta, boiled potatoes, French fries
- Protein-rich foods: cheddar cheese, poached eggs, boiled lentils, baked beans, beefsteak, whitefish
- Breakfast cereals: Cornflakes, Special K, Honeysnacks, Sustain, All-Bran, natural muesli, oatmeal porridge
- Snack foods with confectionery: Mars Bar, strawberry yogurt, vanilla ice cream, jellybeans, salted roasted peanuts, plain potato crisps, plain popcorn
- Bakery products: croissant, chocolate cake with icing, doughnuts with cinnamon sugar, chocolate chip cookies, water crackers

The individual food's capacity to create a feeling of fullness, or satiety, in each participant was studied. On the basis of the study's results, Holt established what she called a *satiety index*, or a rating system that determined each food's ability to create a feeling of fullness on a specific number of calories.

Not surprisingly, the foods that had the least capacity to fill people up were foods that were rich in fat and sugar. The study participants had to eat more of these foods in order to feel full. The foods that created the greatest feeling of fullness were natural plant foods, especially fruit and the starchy carbohydrate-rich foods (with the exception of French fries, which are loaded with fat and have no fiber). By far, the most filling food was the potato, followed closely by oatmeal.

Any time the study participants ate a food that contained both fat and sugar, they found that the food was especially weak at satisfying hunger. Thus, the least satiating food group was the bakery products, and among those foods, the least satiating was the croissant, which contains both fat (butter) and sugar. Croissants were followed by (in order of increasing satiety): cake with icing, doughnuts, cookies, and crackers. The irony, of course, is that these foods are loaded with calories, yet they provide the least satiety, calorie for calorie, when compared to plant foods.

Another group that provided very poor satiety was the snacks and confectionery, another set of foods that have "concentrated" calories, thanks to the presence of either fat or sugar—or both. The food that provided the least satiety among the snacks was the Mars Bar (which contains fat and sugar), followed by peanuts (which contain fat), yogurt (which contains both fat and sugar), potato chips (also rich in fat), ice cream (loaded with fat and sugar), jellybeans (rich in sugar), and popcorn.

Although no food studied by Holt surpasses the potato for its ability to fill you up, fruit was the group of foods that created the greatest feelings of fullness. Oranges were the most filling of the fruits, followed by apples, grapes, and bananas (the least filling fruit). Carbohydrate-rich foods were next on the satiety-index. After the potato, the foods that provided the greatest satiety were brown pasta, whole-meal bread, white rice, brown rice, white pasta, and, least filling of all, French fries (which, of course, have fat).

Of the protein foods, fish was the most filling, followed by steak.

In general, foods that contained fiber and water provided the greatest satiety. Fiber and water provide bulk, which fills you up. At the same time, fiber and water have no calories, which means that you experience fullness, without gaining weight. Of course, the food group with the highest fiber and water content, and the least fat and sugar, is vegetables. These foods were not even studied by Holt because 250 calories of them would be more than most people could eat at a single meal.

Clearly, different foods create very different feelings of fullness. But most of us already know this, if not consciously then intuitively. We know that once we start eating French fries or potato chips, we want to eat more. "Bet you can't eat just one" was more than an effective advertising slogan. It reflects a deep understanding of human nature, which is why the ad is so effective. Not only does it tell the truth, but it tempts you to go out and buy potato chips. The question is: Why? Why can't we eat "just one," and why, after seeing a bag of potato chips or ice cream or a hamburger do so many of us want to buy those foods?

Is this some quirky little characteristic of human nature, an Achilles' heel that Mother Nature gave us to make us fat and unhealthy? Or is there some significance behind our desire for fat, and our capacity to eat so much of it at a single sitting?

In fact, this little quirk of ours doesn't really make sense until you understand the fat instinct. Then the slogan "Bet you can't eat just one" becomes a doorway into the depths of human nature.

UNDER THE SPELL OF AN UNCONTROLLABLE INSTINCT

The fat instinct has America and much of the western world in its grip. Like a demon that possesses its host, the fat instinct lies dormant within all of us much of the time, awaiting its moment to overtake our consciousness and direct our actions. The instant it is triggered, it asserts an overwhelming craving for high-fat, high-calorie foods—and lots of them. For most of us, discipline alone is useless against it. I say "most of us" because about 5 percent of the population—a group of people called "restrained eaters"—can do it. They can control their eating while they endure all the discomforts. The rest of us can't do it. The reason is simple: The fat instinct is a basic and essential part of our will to survive. Using discipline to overcome the fat instinct is like using your willpower to control your desire to breathe. Try taking only short breaths for a while. It's going to require lots of concentration and effort, and eventually your discipline is going to snap and you're going to start binge breathing. There's a limit to how much you will fight to accomplish your own death.

TOO MUCH TEMPTATION

Part of the reason why fatty foods are so hard to avoid is that our fat instinct has given rise to a vast food industry that profits by catering to it. If you drive down any major thoroughfare in the United States, you're assaulted by the riotous colors of fast-food restaurants. Each one shouts for your attention and reminds you that fast food is really fast fat. Thus, a simple drive to the grocery store or the post office is a ride down temptation lane. It is as arousing to your fat instinct as the same ride would be to your libido if American highways were lined with pleasure palaces. Indeed, the fat instinct may even be stronger than your sex drive, because your desire for fat is tied more immediately to your instinct to survive.

Today, our craving for fat is causing our destruction. Excessive consumption of fat is a primary cause of cardiovascular disease, adult-onset diabetes, overweight, many forms of cancer, and other degenerative illnesses. Cardiovascular disease afflicts more than sixty million Americans and accounts for 40 percent of all deaths. Cancer kills more than a half million Americans each year. Currently, more than thirteen million suffer from type II or adult-onset diabetes. More than half of Americans are overweight, and nearly a third are obese. Certain dietary fats are essential; these are needed only in small doses. However, excess fat can be lethal. In fact, fat in large quantities is the greatest toxin in the food supply; yet it is also the food we have been trained by nature to prefer.

Where Is It All Leading?

In *On the Origin of Species* (1859), Charles Darwin addressed the question of what happens when a species suddenly is made to live under environmental conditions that are vastly different from those under which it evolved: "We know that species which have long been exposed to nearly uniform conditions, when they are subjected under confinement to new and greatly changed conditions, either perish, or if they survive, are rendered sterile. . . ."

Today, humans face an epidemic of disease that flows from a dramatic change in their environmental conditions, namely a diet and lifestyle vastly different from the one on which they evolved. Ironically, the genetics we have developed over thousands of years to increase our chances of survival now appear to be the greatest threat to our health and longevity. Because we do not understand the fat instinct, all the current programs designed to create weight loss pit discipline against mother nature—and discipline doesn't have a chance of winning that battle.

REJECTED MIRACLES

WE HAVE THE ANSWERS TO THE MODERN PLAGUE

Sixty million Americans suffer today from cardiovascular disease, or illnesses of the heart and arteries. Each year, more than one million Americans are diagnosed with cancer; if you include nonmalignant skin cancers, which are typically omitted from cancer statistics, the number of new cancers diagnosed annually are two million. By the year 2000, cancer could be the leading cause of death in the country. Meanwhile, thirteen million Americans have adult-onset diabetes. Twenty-five million suffer from osteoporosis, or porous bones. More than one hundred million are overweight, with more than 25 percent of them obese.

The solution to most of these illnesses already exists. Scientists know with certainty that the vast majority of these diseases are preventable with appropriate diet and exercise. The problem we face is that we do not want to take the medicine. Our society, in effect, has rejected the solution. Instead, we adopt every new fad diet that comes along, hoping it can save us from having to adopt the diet we were designed to eat.

That solution wasn't known back in the 1950s, when my father contracted heart disease. He had been following the literature on heart disease, cancer, adult-onset diabetes, and other illnesses since the early 1940s, and he suspected that all of these disorders—including overweight—were somehow linked. Later on, he would discover that they all have the same underlying cause.

Not only did he believe that diet caused disease, but he also felt certain that appropriate diet could cure it. That was a pretty big leap in 1958, but in fact there was enough scientific evidence to suggest vaguely that certain foods and behaviors promoted human health, while others caused life-threatening diseases. My father was counting on his ability to take the few available clues, put them together into a coherent picture, and figure out the mystery of heart disease.

In many ways, he was a scientific detective, and like Sam Spade or Philip Marlowe he had no allegiances once he was on a case. If he had discovered that a diet made up exclusively of lentil beans or steak could save his life, he would have eaten either one of these foods for breakfast, lunch, and dinner. It was with that kind of rigorous commitment that he searched for the healing diet. He left no clue unexamined, and spared himself no discomfort.

He made up extensive charts on which he would enter his blood and urinalysis records. He then underwent an extensive series of tests to obtain his baseline values. For the next ten years, he monitored more than fifty blood constituents, including his total cholesterol, red and white blood cell counts, hemoglobin, proteins, platelets, lactic acid, and virtually every nutrient. His urinalysis was also detailed. Then he began making dramatic changes in his diet, which he monitored with regular blood and urine tests to see what effects, if any, the dietary changes had on his health.

Some of his dietary changes were essentially fasts. In June 1958, he ate little else but lentil beans for weeks. He followed the lentil bean diet with the all-beef diet, which he maintained for a couple more weeks. The beef diet was followed by the brown rice diet, which was followed by the fruit diet. His notes reveal how carefully he kept track of the foods he was eating. "Eating 10 dates after dinner," he noted in one entry. "Start fruit at 1,000 calories, 55 percent total intake," says another. "Three weeks on fruit at 55 to 60 percent total calories, 1,000–1,200 calories fruit," he wrote later on.

Meanwhile, he monitored his blood and urinalysis, paying special attention to his cholesterol level. Today, the words *blood cholesterol* are part of the standard lexicon of westerners. We all have good reason to be concerned about cholesterol because we know that dietary fat and cholesterol raise blood cholesterol and give rise to atherosclerosis, heart attacks, and strokes. High cholesterol is even a major risk factor in cancer. But in 1958, the words *blood cholesterol* were essentially irrelevant to doctors, and meant nothing to laypeople. Nevertheless, my father had seen its importance and started to investigate the effects of individual foods on his cholesterol level.

In 1959, just three years before his diagnosis of heart disease, his blood records reveal that his cholesterol level was 280 mg/dl. He often said that his cholesterol was routinely at 300 mg/dl before his coronary disease was diagnosed. After the lentil bean diet, his cholesterol level fell to 102 mg/dl. It went up sharply to 158 mg/dl when he added beef to his diet, and fell again to 118 mg/dl when he went back to grains, vegetables, beans, fruit and an occasional piece of fish. Clearly, the vegetable-based diet lowered his blood cholesterol substantially, but once he went back to meat his cholesterol started to climb again.

Not only did he monitor the effects on his blood and urine, but he also kept track of any symptoms he experienced during these changes. In January 1969, he wrote: "22 days on dried fruit, 12 dates, 60 percent calories on dried fruit; calories 1,800, was thirsty last two weeks, constant dry taste in mouth."

Over the course of a decade, he would periodically make these fast-like dietary changes, taking breaks from his normal diet of grains, vegetables, beans, fruit, and low-fat animal foods, the diet he decided early on would be best for him, based on the available evidence.

Meanwhile, his doctors thought that his search for a healing diet was ridiculous. Throughout the fifties and sixties, they repeatedly asserted that not only couldn't he cure his heart disease—medical science maintained that the disease was incurable—but if he remained on his diet, he would experience nutrient deficiencies. He couldn't possibly get enough calcium, iron, or protein on the diet he was on, his physicians maintained. Of course, this criticism concerned my father, a layman with two years of college, because it came from medical doctors who had considerable education and experience. On the other hand, the literature pointed out that plant foods alone contain an abundance of all the essential vitamins and minerals—including calcium and iron—as well as optimal amounts of protein. The only exceptions were vitamins B_{12} and D. Vitamin B_{12} is found only in animal foods, but since he ate fish, he had no trouble getting enough B_{12}. Vitamin D can be made in the skin when exposed to sunlight. The body requires only twenty minutes of sunlight per day on your hands and face to produce enough vitamin D. Besides, vitamin D is fat soluble and stored in the fat cells of the body. Thus, as far as my father could tell, nutrient deficiencies shouldn't be a problem, at least in theory. Nevertheless, he kept close track of his blood levels of essential vitamins and minerals as he carried out his dietary experiments.

Eight years after he began his program, an extensive series of tests, including EKG and stress treadmill, revealed that my father had done something that medical science had said was impossible: he had cured himself of heart disease. Moreover, throughout the ten years he experimented with his diet—and indeed, throughout the thirty years that he followed what became known as the Pritikin diet—he never had any nutrient deficiency. We now know that, if anything, a plant-based diet will cause blood nutrient levels to rise.

"It really was not that complicated," he told audiences many years later. "After a couple of months, I realized I was no different than any of the animal studies. The same way animals drop their cholesterol level [after going on a vegetable-based diet], so do humans. I never did run into deficiencies, or have any problems at all with getting adequate nutrition. I was just frightened unnecessarily."

In the course of his research, he found that a high-fat diet not only is a major cause of heart disease, but also contributes to many other degenerative diseases, including cancer, adult-onset diabetes, high blood pressure, and overweight. In effect, the modern diet is poisoning us. Our genetic makeup causes us to be more susceptible to one disease or another, which is why one person who eats a high-fat diet gets heart disease, while others get cancer, or diabetes, or some other degenerative disease.

This discovery becomes more relevant every day because our society now places so much hope in genetic research's ability to provide the answers to disease. Implicit within the findings of the modern research, and certainly consistent with what my father discovered, is the fact that you can have a genetic predisposition to an illness that may never materialize unless you create the right conditions for those genes to be expressed. A diet rich in fat and cholesterol will increase the likelihood that whatever genetic weakness you have will manifest as an illness. On the other hand, you can prevent the expression of those genes by avoiding the dietary excesses that ultimately expose your genetic weakness.

Once my father found that diet was both a primary cause of and the cure for many illnesses, he began to consider an interesting question. Why would certain foods cause illness, while others improve health? This question led him to believe that *perhaps there is a diet that humans are designed to eat, one that promotes health and protects us from most diseases.*

Logic pointed directly to such a possibility, since a major part of our evolution included the process by which human biology adapted to the foods that were available in our environment. Certain foods dominated the diets of our ancestors. The challenge early humans faced was to adapt biologically so that they could extract the maximum amounts of nutrition from these foods, and thereby survive. Over millions of years, the foods that made up that diet, in effect, shaped our organs, the chemical function of our livers, even the digestive enzymes in our mouth. As David Attenborough described in his book *Life on Earth*, nature used food as one of the tools to design us.

In fact, the human body's physical makeup—its nutritional needs and biochemical strengths and limitations—is now sufficiently understood to determine the kinds of foods and nutrients it needs. Scientists today know that the diet we evolved on is made up largely of plant foods, such as vegetables, beans, grains, and fruit, coupled with relatively smaller quantities of animal foods, such as meat, eggs, and poultry. As I showed in chapter 1, this diet was extremely low in fat, because even the animal foods our ancestors ate were lean.

Now, I know what many people are thinking: How can anyone be sure that we are designed to eat certain foods more than others? After all, the so-called experts are making vastly conflicting statements about what is best for us to eat. Some say we should eat lots of meat, eggs, and dairy, in other words, a high-protein diet. Others advocate vegetarianism. Who can say what is true?

To paraphrase the great detective Sherlock Holmes, "If you study the clues and, on the basis of those clues, eliminate all the possibilities but one, what you have left is the truth."

THE HUMAN DIET

What we're looking for is a diet that is nutritionally much closer to that of our ancestors, the diet that shaped their biological and genetic makeup, and our own. There are three types of evidence that scientists can study to discover that diet. The first is fossil evidence, which in this case is primarily copralite, or the petrified feces of our ancestors. The second is anatomical. The human body has a specific design that can be compared with that of other species known to be plant eaters, such as rabbits or horses, and those that are meat eaters, such as cats. The third form of evidence is biochemical. Our bodies have very specific needs for vitamins and minerals. We also have limited abilities to cope with chronically high levels of fat, particularly saturated fat, which must be respected if we are to avoid disease. All of this evidence points to the kind of diet on which we evolved, and the one on which the body still runs best.

Fossils

Copralite dates back to a time when early humans were roaming the forests of Africa. By looking at the spent fuel of a machine, you can tell a lot about the fuel that machine consumed. Pioneering researchers Denis Burkitt and Hugh Trowell spent twenty-five years in the African wilderness examining the health patterns of Africans, and unearthing evidence of our ancient forebears. What they found was that the fossilized feces of early humans contain exceedingly high levels of fiber, indicating a diet made up predominantly of plant foods, with smaller amounts of animal foods.

Other researchers, including Konner and Eaton, agree with this assessment. They maintain that even among early hunter-gatherer tribes, vegetable foods made up anywhere from 65 to 80 percent of the Paleolithic diet, which would provide at least 50 to 100 grams or more of fiber per day, compared to only 10 to 15 grams that the average American consumes each day.

Dr. Adrienne Zihlman, a professor of anthropology at the University of California at Santa Cruz, points out that if early humans had to rely primarily upon animal foods to support their daily need for nutrition and calories, we would have died out long ago. There simply was not enough animal food to feed women, children, and the men who remained at home while other men scavenged, sometimes for days and weeks at a time. This explains why the petrified feces of our ancestors reveal a high-fiber diet.

Daily survival depended on the foods most available, which were plants. And when it comes to the most efficient use of time and energy, the gathering of plant foods is a whole lot easier and quicker than hunting, killing, and slaughtering an animal, notes Dr. A. S. Truswell of the Department of Nutrition and Food Science at the University of London. Truswell and others have studied the !Kung of Botswana, a people who maintain their traditional diet and ways of living, many of which date back to Paleolithic times. As Truswell points out, it takes the !Kung women four hours to gather 1,000 calories of plant foods; it takes the men ten hours to return home with the caloric equivalent in meat.

Our dependence on fruits and vegetables has existed for millions of years, and consequently has shaped our genetic makeup. In the process, it has given rise to the anatomic structure of modern humans.

Anatomy: A Herbivore's Design

Like other plant eaters—both herbivores and omnivores—we have jaws that are capable of both vertical and horizontal movement. This allows us to thoroughly grind fibrous foods. The jaws of carnivores like cats are quite different. They are capable of vertical movements only, which is all that's needed when you have to bite down and tear flesh.

Human saliva is very different chemically from that of carnivores. A carnivore's saliva is acidic. Human saliva, like that of herbivores, is alkaline and contains the enzyme amylase, which starts the digestion of the starches that are found almost exclusively in plant-based foods.

We also have long, meandering digestive tracts, another common trait of herbivores and omnivores. Carnivores, on the other hand, have short digestive tracts, designed to eliminate meat rapidly.

Long digestive tracts such as ours are needed to break down fibrous plant foods and extract the nutrients from them, especially the carbohydrates that are bound up inside the fiber. This is a difficult and time-consuming task. A long digestive tract permits food to remain within the small intestine long enough for the body to extract the nutrients from fiber-based foods. Though the fiber slows the extraction of nutrition within the small intestine, it also speeds the elimination of waste from the large intestine, or colon.

When we eat a diet that is low in fiber and high in meat and fat, we stress our digestive system. The absence of fiber prevents efficient elimination and promotes the onset of constipation, diverticulosis, hemorrhoids, and even colon cancer.

The Biochemical Evidence

Of all the nutrients the human body requires, fewer than fifty cannot be produced by the body itself, and therefore must be obtained from dietary sources. Of that fifty, forty-eight are found in abundance in vegetable foods. The forty-ninth, vitamin D, comes from sunlight, and the fiftieth, vitamin B_{12}, is obtained from animal sources only. Interestingly, we have developed the ability to store vitamin B_{12} for five to seven years before we need to consume another round of animal flesh in order to replenish our supply of the vitamin. We may have developed that ability because the availability of animal foods was unpredictable.

Finally, there is the problem of metabolizing cholesterol. Diets high in saturated fat, hydrogenated fat, and cholesterol impair the liver's ability to remove cholesterol from the blood. Like all other animal cells, human cells produce cholesterol, a chemical that's used to make many hormones and vitamin D, and maintain healthy cellular membranes. Only the tissues of animals have cholesterol. All vegetables are 100 percent cholesterol-free. We generate all the cholesterol our bodies need, which means that we do not have to get any cholesterol from food. Rabbits and other purely vegetarian species have limited ability to process dietary cholesterol safely, and thus rapidly develop atherosclerosis and heart disease when they consume cholesterol-containing foods. Cats and other carnivores are able to respond physiologically to their dietary cholesterol by drawing excess cholesterol into their livers and excreting it through the intestines. At the same time, carnivores are able to reduce their body's cholesterol production to compensate for the cholesterol they consume. Thus, cats can eat all the cholesterol-rich foods they want, such as birds, eggs, and rodents, without any negative side effects.

Unfortunately, humans do not have a carnivore's ability to rid the body of cholesterol. Our livers have a very limited capacity to draw cholesterol out of the blood and safely eliminate it. That means that the more cholesterol we eat, the more disease we suffer. This is not to say that we cannot process cholesterol; it's just that our ability is limited.

It must be remembered that our ancestors were rarely able to get much fat in their diets, even when they were eating meat. Our ancestors ate animals that were raised in the wild, which meant that the animal flesh they did eat was extremely low in fat. As Konner and Eaton point out, the animals in the wild have an average fat content of about 3.9 percent—a low-fat food under any circumstances!

We are omnivores, but with a catch. We must strictly limit the amount of animal foods we eat; otherwise, they poison us.

After studying the health and dietary patterns of 6,500 Chinese living in China, Dr. T. Colin Campbell, a nutritionist and biochemist at Cornell University, found that the best predictor of whether or not a Chinese person would suffer a serious illness was his or her blood cholesterol level.

"So far we've seen that plasma cholesterol is a good predictor of the kinds of diseases people are going to get," Dr. Campbell told the New York Times. "Those with higher cholesterol levels are prone to diseases of affluence—cancer, heart disease, and diabetes. . . . We're basically a vegetarian species and should be eating a wide variety of plant foods and minimizing our intake of animal foods."

The bottom line is that anatomists, anthropologists, archeologists, and nutritionists all concur that the most healthful human diet is dominated by plant foods, with varying amounts of low-fat animal foods. Our Paleolithic ancestors ate at least three times more plant foods than we do today, and the animal foods they ate were anywhere from two to six times lower in fat than the animal foods we eat today. When our ancestors sat down to a "high-fat" meal and really gorged on all the fat-calories they could get, they were still eating a "low-fat" meal by modern standards.

TRADITIONAL SOCIETIES

Traditional peoples fascinated my father. He recognized that traditional peoples hold the secrets to our ancient past and our evolution as humans (whether the aborigines of Australia, the Highlanders of New Guinea, the !Kung of Botswana, the Bantus of South Africa, or the native peoples of the Americas). Many traditional peoples still maintain the diets and lifestyles that are very similar—if not identical—to those of our Paleolithic ancestors. If you want to know how humans function on the traditional diet, all you have to do is examine the disease patterns of these people. Indeed, to study traditional cultures is to go back in time to discover the secrets of our own biological nature.

My father held on to that idea and used it like a compass on his journey through the mysteries of health. Whenever a new dietary program or practice was being touted as the latest answer to our health concerns, he would wonder aloud if anyone in the world actually lived according to that idea. Do humans have any experience with such foods or ways of living? he would ask. If the answer was yes, we could investigate the effects of such a diet or lifestyle on human health. If the answer was no, then the idea was merely a concept that needed long-term study. In any case, we would know that a diet consistently high in fat was probably foreign to our evolution and therefore foreign to our biology. It would take a very long time to make it fit with our anatomy, he realized.

Given his love for traditional cultures, it was no wonder that among my father's favorite books was one of the preeminent works of anthropology, *The Golden Bough* (1890), by Sir James Frazer. Frazer, a Scottish anthropologist and classicist, examined the roots of religious thinking in primitive societies around the world, and linked such belief systems to modern institutions and ways of living. Recently, I was paging through the updated version of Frazer's book, *The New*

Golden Bough, revised by renowned scholar Theodor H. Gaster, Ph.D. As I read the book, I marveled at the reverence traditional peoples paid to whole, unprocessed grain. Grain kept the people alive and healthy, and therefore was conceived of in religious and mythological terms. Among Native Americans, rituals were performed each season to sustain the fertility of the soil and give thanks for the ongoing blessing of the "Corn Mother," as they referred to the deity who provided their people with their most sacred food.

My father had no special interest in the specific mythologies each society attached to their agriculture—but he was fascinated by their recognition of grain and vegetables as the source of health and longevity. Primitive people recognized that human existence hung by a few tenuous threads, one of which was cultivated vegetables.

In fact, the American Indians said as much. They maintained that the Corn Mother had provided them with a grain that was easily cultivated, yielded abundant supplies of food, and kept them healthy and alive with little effort. But the Indians had a legend about their dependence on corn that would prove prophetic as well as tragic. They maintained that corn would be the basis of their civilization until the day came when the people would be struck by a great evil that would blight the fields and destroy the purity of the corn. For the Pima Indians of Arizona, that dark day came around 1900. They have never recovered.

The Pimas—and the Fork in the Road

The Pima Indians are descendants of migrating Asians who, perhaps thirty thousand years ago, crossed the Bering Straits and eventually settled in the desert of what is now Arizona and northwest Mexico. When the Spanish explorers arrived in these lands, they called the four-hundred-mile swath of land that ran from the Gila and Salt Rivers (now Arizona) to the Sierra Madre Mountains (today the Mexican state of Sonora) "Pimeria."

The Arizona Pimas developed a sophisticated knowledge of agriculture and irrigation, turning the arid desert into fertile gardens by channeling the water of the Gila River into their fields, where they raised corn, beans, squash, and a variety of other vegetables. They supplemented their diets with small amounts of fish and game that lived close to the rivers.

Here, the Pimas thrived for thousands of years on their simple diets and traditional ways. But all of that changed in 1900 when white settlers from the East diverted the water from the rivers and turned the Piman gardens into an empty desert. The Pimas tried to hold on to their traditional life, but over the next two generations their simple ways of eating and living were destroyed. Eventually, they became dependent on surplus food issued by the U.S. government, the most abundant of which were animal foods loaded with fat and cholesterol. A people who once thrived on a diet of complex carbohydrates from unprocessed corn, beans, squash, and vegetables now were forced to live on a diet that derived more than 40 percent of its calories from fat. The effects of such a diet on the Pimas were devastating.

In the 1950s, the Pimas started to develop widespread obesity and non-insulin-dependent diabetes mellitus (NIDDM). The onset of these diseases happened suddenly. Obesity and diabetes spread through the Piman population like a forest fire. Today, the Pima Indians suffer from the highest rates of obesity and diabetes of any people on earth. More than a third of their women (37 percent) and more than half of the men (54 percent) have diabetes. Most Pimas develop severe obesity, often in childhood, and by the age of fifty most have diabetes as well. That means that they spend the rest of their lives coping with these illnesses and the many disorders they give rise to.

Diabetes is like a bad tree with many virulent branches, each one a life-altering disorder. In fact, rarely do diabetics suffer from diabetes alone. The illness predisposes its sufferers to exceedingly high rates of kidney failure, blindness, claudication, gangrene, and the loss of limbs. Not surprisingly, the Pimas spend much of their lives suffering, and many die young.

This is what the modern diet and lifestyle have wrought among the Pima Indians—or at least one branch of the Piman family. Recently, scientists learned of another branch living in a remote part of the Sierra Madre Mountains in northwest Mexico. These Mexican Pimas have spent their lives away from the big cities of Mexico and the United States. Their village got its first paved road in 1992; before that, they were linked with the capitals of Sonora and Chihuahua by dirt roads that could be traversed only by horse-drawn carts or four-wheel-drive vehicles. Because of their relative inaccessibility, the Mexican Pimas have maintained their traditional diets and ways of living, and consequently have kept their health.

The Mexican Pimas live primarily on corn tortillas, beans, squash, rice, potatoes, pasta soups, and a narrow variety of other vegetables. They drink coffee and soda pop (when they can get it), eat eggs occasionally, and fry their beans in small amounts of vegetable oils. They rarely eat red meat and poultry. According to researcher Eric Ravussin, Ph.D., and his colleagues who compared the diets and health patterns of thirty-five Mexican Pimas with a matched group of Arizona Pimas, the Mexican Pimas eat meat and chicken once every month or two. With the high concentration of grains and beans, they consume more than 50 grams of fiber per day. Overall, Dr. Ravussin and his coworkers determined that the diet of Mexican Pimas is composed of 63 percent complex carbohydrates, 13 percent protein, 23 percent fat (mostly of vegetable origin), and less than 1 percent alcohol.

As you might expect, the Mexican Pimas work hard, and their lifestyles are reflected in their health patterns. Most of the men are farmers, wood mill and construction workers, cowboys, and fence builders. The women work at home and in the family gardens.

Unlike the Arizona Pimas, the Mexican Pimas are lean and relatively disease-free. In fact, there was no comparison between the two branches of the Piman family. As Dr. Ravussin and his group showed, each Mexican Pima is, on average, fifty-seven pounds lighter than his or her Arizona Pima counterpart. Mexican Pimas are much more muscular and have a much lower percentage of body fat. The Mexican Pimas have far lower blood cholesterol levels (more than thirty points lower, on average), and diabetes is rare among the Mexican Pimas.

The Mexican Pimas are strong and vital right up to old age; the Arizona Pimas are weak and diseased, often starting very young in life. The Mexican Pimas require very little medical care, while the Arizona Pimas require constant medical intervention, much of which becomes highly invasive, frightening, and painful, especially as the Arizona men and women grow older.

Interestingly, researchers point out that all Pima Indians—whether they come from Mexico or Arizona—probably have the same genetic susceptibility to obesity and diabetes. Yet, only the Pimas of Arizona get these diseases because only the Arizona Pimas maintain a lifestyle that will bring out, or cause the expression of, their genetic predisposition. The reason the Mexican Pimas are protected is simple: they eat a diet that is low in fat and cholesterol and rich in unprocessed complex carbohydrates. At the same time, they maintain a way of life that includes physical activity, which is consistent with the lifestyle on which their ancestors evolved. The diet and lifestyle even protect the Mexican Pimas against diseases for which there is a genetic predisposition. Yes, genes do play a role in the susceptibility to develop certain diseases, but genetic weakness is the most misunderstood and overused rationalization for explaining why we currently suffer from epidemics of degenerative illnesses. Potential for disease is not a guarantee. The right environmental factors can protect against the onset of many major illnesses, including certain types of cancer, heart disease, type II or adult-onset diabetes, overweight, and high blood pressure. On the other hand, the consumption of high-fat and high-calorie foods can increase the likelihood that a genetic weakness will be expressed, thus causing one or another of these serious illnesses to manifest.

Rural vs. Urban Asian Diets

The Pimas are by no means unique in this regard. The same phenomenon occurs among many traditional peoples throughout the world as their diets and lifestyles become westernized. For many years, researchers suspected that the Japanese had a genetic protection against the illnesses associated with western culture, namely heart disease and the common cancers, those of the breast, prostate, and colon. But when Japanese immigrated to the United States and adopted the standard American diet, they began to suffer from the same diseases as other Americans: high levels of cardiovascular disease, cancer, diabetes, and other degenerative disorders.

Dr. T. Colin Campbell and his colleagues at Cornell University studied sixty-five hundred people from sixty-five geographical counties of China (one hundred people from each county). As you might expect, the dietary habits of people vary dramatically based on whether they lived in big cities or rural environments. Not surprisingly, the disease patterns correlate to the amount of fat and cholesterol these people ate. Those Chinese who maintain the traditional Chinese diet—composed chiefly of rice, vegetables, and small amounts of fish—have extremely low rates of the diseases common in the West, such as heart disease, cancer, type II or adult-onset diabetes, and obesity, while those who eat a diet similar to that of westerners have the same disease patterns as Americans do.

The rural Chinese actually eat slightly more calories than Americans do, but most of their calories come from vegetable foods. Consequently, they are lean and obesity is rare. They also eat about 60 percent less fat than we do and a third less protein. Not only do they eat less protein, but they get most of their protein from plants. Seventy percent of Americans' protein comes from animal sources, such as red meat, dairy foods, and eggs, while only 7 percent of the protein in the Chinese diet comes from animal sources. As you might expect, the Chinese have very low cholesterol levels, averaging 127 mg/dl of blood. Adult Americans average 210 mg/dl.

Are the Chinese immune to the diseases Americans commonly suffer? No. When Chinese people move to their country's big cities, or emigrate and adopt western diets, they develop many of the same diseases. Their primary form of protection must be their traditional diet and lifestyle, which is much closer to our ancestors'.

All of this research points to a rather startling fact about this wondrous machine, the human body. It was designed to enjoy good health, abundant energy, and long life. Except in the case of an accident contagion, or genetic disorder, you were never intended to become dependent on medical doctors, or drugs, or even require an operation, except perhaps in very old age. Many people point to our life expectancy as a source of pride in our technology and medical understanding, but the !Kung of Botswana have the same percentage of people older than sixty in their society as Americans do. And if a member of the !Kung community doesn't die from an accident or an infection early in life, he or she has a better chance of living to a ripe old age than you and I do. Yet, the !Kung receive no medical treatment throughout their lives.

You were designed to run perfectly for a very long time. The way to enjoy the good health that is your birthright is simple: eat the foods that you were designed to eat and maintain an active life. In exchange, you can have optimal health, energy, and long life. When you think about it, that's not really a bad deal.

THE PRITIKIN TRACK RECORD

At the Pritikin Longevity Center, we have witnessed the power of the traditional human diet to restore health, even after only a few weeks on our regimen. We have been using that diet, along with a program of moderate exercise, for the past twenty years to treat more than sixty-five thousand people suffering from a wide array of degenerative diseases, including overweight, coronary heart disease, angina, high blood pressure, and adult-onset diabetes. Scientific analyses have reported our dramatic results in the scientific and medical literature, as well as the lay press. Here are just a few of the revelations scientists have reported:

Cholesterol and Triglycerides Levels

Research has shown that the average drop in blood cholesterol among people who come to our centers and adopt our program is 23 percent; the average drop in triglycerides, or blood fats, is 33 percent.

High Blood Pressure

Of those studied who came to our center with high blood pressure and who were taking medication, fully 83 percent left with normal blood pressure and free of any need for pharmaceutical drugs.

Angina and Candidates for Bypass Surgery

A study examining a group of patients who were scheduled to have bypass surgery but came to the Pritikin Longevity Center instead showed that 80 percent of these people did not need the surgery after adopting our program. Five years later, they still didn't need the surgery.

Adult-Onset Diabetes

A study of people with adult-onset diabetes who were taking insulin found that 39 percent left our center with normal blood sugar levels and off all insulin. Of those adult-onset diabetics who came to our center taking oral medication, 70 percent no longer needed their diabetes drugs when they left.

Breast and Colon Cancer Risk Factors

When scientists examined the major risk factors for breast and colon cancer, they found that people who adopted the Pritikin Program reduced several of those risk factors by as much as 50 percent.

No medically supervised diet and health program available can duplicate the results the Pritikin Program has demonstrated over the past two decades. At our centers we use a diet nutritionally similar to the one humans evolved on to get these results. When a diet similar to ours is applied to populations who suffer from modern degenerative diseases such as overweight and adult-onset diabetes, research has shown that the health of these people is restored. Consider the case of the native Hawaiians.

RESTORING THE HAWAIIAN TRADITIONAL DIET— AND HAWAIIAN HEALTH

When you think of Hawaii, you think of tropical islands, sunshine, palm trees, sandy beaches, and big waves. If you look at some health statistics you find that, on average, Hawaii has the highest life expectancy of any state in the union. But Hawaii has a dark side, too. Native Hawaiians, or the people of Asian descent who first came to the Islands thousands of years ago, have the lowest life expectancy of any ethnic group in the country. One of the primary reasons for their short life span is that by middle age they are almost uniformly obese. Only the Pima Indians have a higher rate of obesity, but the Pimas live longer on average than the native Hawaiians do because they appear to be genetically less susceptible to coronary heart disease.

Historical accounts of nineteenth-century Hawaiians report that these native people were generally thin and healthy, but all that changed when the native population dropped their traditional diet and adopted the modern, high-fat, high-cholesterol regimen that caused obesity and cardiovascular disease to skyrocket among them.

In 1990 a group of researchers led by Dr. Terry T. Shintani got twenty native Hawaiians to adopt their traditional diet for twenty-one days, during which time the researchers kept track of the study participants' weight, cholesterol levels, and blood pressure. The results were startling.

The diet the Hawaiians adopted derived only 7 percent of its calories from fat, which is what the Hawaiians were used to eating before the middle of this century. Seventy-eight percent of their calories came from complex carbohydrates, and 15 percent from protein. Specifically, the primary foods were taro potato, poi mashed potato (a dish made with taro potato), sweet potato, yams, breadfruit, greens, fruit, seaweed, fish, and chicken. The food was served steamed or raw in the manner that traditional Hawaiians prepared their meals. Only the portions of the fish and chicken were controlled to their traditional amounts. All the other foods were available in unlimited quantities, and the participants were encouraged to eat as much as they wanted.

After the twenty-one days, the average weight loss was more than seventeen pounds. Total blood cholesterol and LDL cholesterol both dropped significantly. Systolic pressure (the pressure created when the heart is contracting) was reduced by 11.5 mm Hg, while diastolic pressure (the pressure created by the arteries when the heart is expanding) dropped 8.9 mm Hg. In other words, the Hawaiians experienced a tremendous improvement in health. They lost nearly twenty pounds in three weeks, yet never experienced hunger! In addition, they significantly reduced their risk of heart attack, stroke, cancer, and adult-onset diabetes. No pill or potion could do for these people what their traditional way of eating did in less than a month. The problem was, they were still driven by the fat instinct, which meant that as soon as the researchers stopped the experiment, the Hawaiians went right back to their old high-fat diets.

BREAK THE SPELL OF THE FAT INSTINCT

Here's the dark irony of modern life that reveals just how powerful the fat instinct is: *Science has devoted millions of dollars to finding the diet most beneficial to human health. That diet has been discovered. Yet, no one wants to eat it!* In fact, most of us do everything possible to avoid the diet we were designed to eat.

The vast majority of Americans are no different from the native Hawaiians, Australian aborigines, or Pima Indians. When the Pima Indians were encouraged to go back to their traditional diets, they told the researchers, "no way." The same is true of the Australian aborigines. In fact, one group of researchers actually offered to pay the aborigines to eat their traditional diet in order to document its health effects, but after three months, the aborigines flatly refused to continue—even for twice the money!

On the surface, we all know why Americans, Pima Indians, native Hawaiians, and Australian aborigines would rather enjoy their high-fat diets and be sick than eat the diet that would cure their diseases and give them good health. Simply put, the cure doesn't taste as good as the cause.

Remember the study I reported in chapter 1 done by Susanne Holt and her colleagues? That study demonstrated that high-fat, high-sugar foods provided the lowest satiety, which means that you have to eat more of these foods to create a feeling of fullness. Holt found, however, that these same foods have the greatest palatability.

A little fat and sugar are perfectly acceptable. Dose determines whether or not a food substance becomes a poison. Unfortunately, every time we encounter a high-fat or high-calorie meal, the fat instinct kicks in and makes sure that we either overeat or gorge on these foods.

The fat instinct is alive and well today in each of us. Unless we know how to outsmart it, any confrontation with a high-fat meal will trigger a very powerful set of behaviors that are designed to force you to consume the maximum amount of calories available this very minute. There's no way to avoid the pressure to immediately gratify the fat instinct.

The environment makes unique demands on all of us to adapt and evolve in order to maintain our health. Up until the early part of this century, the fat instinct and our desire for a fit and healthy body were compatible, since the food that was most available to us were plant foods, such as grain, grain products, vegetables, and fruit. In many ways, the ratio of plant and animal foods had not changed all that much since the time of our early ancestors. Remember that as late as 1870, more than half of all Americans (53 percent) worked on farms, which meant that most of their foods were derived from plants. In 1910, between one-third and one-half of all people living in cities were poor. These people could not afford to eat meat on a daily basis; they were lucky if they got it once a week, or twice a month. Even through the thirties and forties, when the Great Depression held sway over the nation's economy, most people didn't have to think about eating too much fat and cholesterol, because such foods were too costly. Thus, the fat instinct was kept at bay by the prevailing environmental and economic forces. These same forces protected us from overweight, obesity, and other disorders that are common today. This meant that the environment was protecting us from disease by limiting the amount of fat that was available to us.

In former times, we didn't have to think about the behaviors that would keep us healthy and keep our fat instinct in check because the environment itself did that for us. In effect, our early ancestors maintained a child-parent relationship with the environment. The environment enforced health-promoting behaviors upon them.

All of that has changed. The supply of fat and high-calorie foods is plentiful, if not limitless, and readily available. At the same time, we still have a very powerful, primitive instinct to eat as much fat as we can lay our hands on. The environment is actually encouraging us to eat foods that can cause widespread disability and death. The fat instinct has gained sway over the western world. This is evident from the high-fat, high-calorie foods we eat, a diet unlike any other in human history, and from the disease patterns and death rates of our times.

Until researchers at the Pritikin Longevity Center uncovered the fat instinct, and how to outsmart and overcome it, most diet-and-health proponents did not fully understand our driving need for fat, or teach us how to conquer it. In the absence of such knowledge, dietary experts tried to teach us how to live with it. Many of today's weight-control programs try to sell you a new version of the high-fat diet, while making it sound like some modern-day equivalent of miracle tonic. The message is: "Yes, you can still have your London broil and your health, too." That's like a drug pusher telling a heroin addict, "You can keep using heroin and still live a normal, healthy life." These programs not only keep you addicted to fat, but also deprive you of the very things you came to the program for in the first place: health, abundant energy, and optimal weight.

It doesn't take us long to figure out that we can't follow these diets for very long and that they can't deliver on their promises. However, there's a new program on the market every year making the same claims, so people end up hopping from one program to the next, with each one ending in failure.

Even people who followed in my father's footsteps now say that healthful eating is not for everyone. Many health proponents believe that a natural diet is no longer for every human, but only for those who are so ill that they're willing to adopt it as a last resort! The fat instinct has created yet another distortion in our thinking and approach to life.

If we stand back and look at this picture from a rational distance, we can see that we are doing everything possible to avoid eating the diet we were designed to eat. We'll try any regimen—high protein, high fat, portion control, and calorie counting. We'll endure hunger and discomfort for weeks. We'll adopt the latest fad diet touting some miraculous nutrient that will answer all of our prayers and let us eat Häagen Dazs, too; we don't care that there's no research to back up its claims. And if all of this fails, as we secretly believe it will, we're even ready to have our chests split open and our coronary arteries bypassed. All this because we don't want to face up to the simple truth that nature designed us to eat primarily starchy foods, fresh vegetables, beans, fruit, and modest amounts of low-fat animal foods. In short, most Americans believe that the cure is worse than the disease.

What we do not realize is that the only thing that stands between each of us and the natural human diet—and good health—is the fat instinct and the environment we have created to keep the fat instinct fed. The fat instinct is in charge, and as long as it is, we're not going to give up eating fat and calorie-rich foods. Until we learn to outsmart the demon within us, we're only going to get fatter and sicker.

WHY DIETING FAILS
IN AMERICA

Right now, fifty million adult Americans are dieting. The reason, obviously, is that we're too fat. More than 60 percent of the adult population in the United States is overweight. There is no shortage of new diets. Americans have more weight-loss programs to choose from than any other people on earth, and new diets appear on the market every year. This is part of the problem. Consumers are inundated with choices, and each one portrays itself as "The New, Revolutionary Approach," the only program on which you can "Eat Your Way to Dynamic Weight Loss." As a long-time observer of the dieting phenomenon, I can tell you with assurance that it will not stop. But do all these programs really offer us a choice?

The truth is that *there are only three ways to lose weight on a diet, no matter what kind of diet you're on.* There hasn't been a new approach to dieting in a very long time. The Pied Pipers have been taking one of these three approaches and dressing it up in new marketing. In most cases, the salesmen behind these diet programs have created a diversion, the way magicians do, to make it seem as if some discovery—a new nutrient, for example—provides the secret to good health and optimal weight. But when it comes to the underlying basic principle used to lose weight, none of them is new. Three thousand years ago, Ecclesiastes offered up some very relevant wisdom. "Vanity of vanities!" said the Preacher. "That which has been done is that which will be done. So, there is nothing new under the sun." In other words, we were warned. What the Preacher didn't say is that the packaging will be different the next time around.

Here are the three approaches that are the basis for all weight-loss diets; (each one has its own set of side effects):

1. *Portion control,* also known as calorie counting or restrained eating. These programs cause weight loss by restricting the amount of food you can eat at each meal. On most portion-control programs, you can eat just about any type of food, as long as you eat only small amounts of it to limit the number of calories you consume. Needless to say, tremendous discipline is needed to lose weight on portion-control diets, because you are constantly hungry, irritable, and tired. Your body is screaming out for food and you've got to suppress that scream.

2. *High-protein, low-carbohydrate diet.* These diets upset your body's metabolism by inducing a state called *ketosis,* in which appetite is suppressed and, initially, lots of water is shed rapidly. The water loss alone causes weight loss. In addition, because the diet diminishes hunger, you eat less food, which means you restrict calories dramatically and lose even more weight. Unfortunately, such diets can have a detrimental impact on your health. In addition, your body craves carbohydrates, its preferred fuel, which prevents people from sticking to such diets for very long. Most high-protein diets are also high in fat and cholesterol, and deficient in the immune-boosting and cancer-fighting substances present in plant foods—chemicals your body needs to sustain health.

3. *Very low-fat, high-fiber diet,* such as the Pritikin diet. This diet is not only the oldest approach on earth to weight loss, but also a tool for preventing most serious illnesses. This is the human diet, the one we were designed to eat, rich in carbohydrates in their natural state, low in fat, and based on vegetables, fruits, unprocessed grains, and low-fat animal foods. Because most of these foods are low in calories, but loaded with bulky fiber, you can eat to satiety and still lose weight. In fact, at the Pritikin Longevity Center we discourage anyone from ever going hungry because hunger triggers the fat instinct, which will awaken your craving for calorie-rich foods and a desire to overeat. The Pritikin Program is designed to outsmart the fat instinct, which is the best way to lose weight and maintain health as you do it. In addition to diet, the Pritikin Program includes moderate exercise (see chapter 6).

PORTION CONTROL: TRIGGERING THE FAT INSTINCT

When Susan, whom we met in chapter 1, began dieting, her primary approach was portion control, or calorie counting. She made no distinction among foods other than their relative calorie content. If she ate a food that contained lots of calories, such as a piece of pie or cake, she couldn't eat much else for the rest of the day, which meant that she was hungry a lot of the time.

Susan didn't realize it, but her calorie-counting diet triggered her fat instinct, unleashing all of its powerful drives and metabolic reactions. The fat instinct was designed by nature to keep us alive in the face of famine. To the hypothalamus, where most of our instinctive behaviors are stored, dieting is just another form of famine. Susan was dieting to lose weight and become more attractive and healthy, but her brain recognized a significant drop in calories as a food shortage and announced, "My life is in danger. Drastic measures are needed."

By now, Susan's fat instinct had entered its second phase, producing an array of symptoms, including hunger pangs, cold extremities, irritability, headache, and physical tension. She also experienced the overpowering urge to eat fat and calorie-rich foods. Pretty soon, Susan found herself craving hamburgers, French fries, cookies, ice cream, and chocolate—any food that was loaded with calories. At this point, the fat instinct is using discomfort alone to drive Susan to eat calorie-rich foods.

Because she is a disciplined person, Susan managed to fight these cravings, maintaining her program even as a host of biological and physiological symptoms got worse. After a while, she lost energy, felt fatigued, and needed to rest as much as possible. She lacked the joie de vivre that was so characteristic of her personality. The burden of hunger was weighing her down.

To Susan, these signals were unexpected. After all, she was eating every day. But she was eating fewer calories than her body was used to consuming. Also, the food she was eating did not provide satiety at this restricted calorie-intake, which only contributed to her desire to eat more food, and her experience of deprivation and hunger.

Dieting is a relatively recent phenomenon in human history. For millions of years, there was only one form of "dieting" and that was starvation. While Susan was saying to herself, "I want to be more attractive; I want my youth and energy back," her body was saying, "I'm starving and dying and you've got to eat in order to keep me alive." Dieting triggered her fat instinct.

Despite the discomforts, Susan's discipline held fast for a time, which was interpreted by her instinctual brain to mean that the famine was continuing. Thus, the famine response was engaged: her body's metabolic rate slowed to conserve calories. Susan's body was doing what evolution has equipped it to do: when food intake declines, the body slows down cellular metabolism to protect energy reserves (mainly in the form of body fat) and, in the process, outlast the famine or food shortage.

In order to maintain Susan's life on fewer calories, Susan's body also discourages any unnecessary activity. She doesn't feel like exercising—even a walk is out of the question—and her ability to work is diminished as well. This need to slow down her activities coordinates perfectly with her metabolic attempts to conserve calories. As far as Susan's body is concerned, exercise is a waste of precious energy. The body can now function more efficiently on the calories Susan is consuming each day. The result is that even though she's starving, she isn't losing a pound.

At this point, the diet has failed, even though Susan's discipline is still holding fast. Her diet has created the conditions in which further weight loss is nearly impossible. In order to lose additional weight, Susan could exercise, but because she feels tired and irritable that's the last thing she wants to do. Or she could eat even less food than she's eating now, which would mean she really would be starving herself. Susan isn't suicidal. Her survival mechanism—and in particular her fat instinct—is healthy and strong, which means that eventually she's going to eat.

Dejected by the fact that she is no longer losing weight and overwhelmed with the sheer misery of dieting, Susan decides to "have a little something to eat." She has been at this juncture several times before with diets, and inevitably that little something turns out to be a hamburger and French fries, or a tuna sandwich with lots of mayonnaise, or even a steak with baked potato and sour cream. At that point, the dam has broken and Susan is gorging.

At this point her lower rate of metabolism really works against her. Since her cells are burning significantly less energy than she's used to, the increase in food—and most of the calories that come with it—will be stored as fat. Susan's going to gain weight because her body is now operating in a way that is conserving calories. In effect, her body's efficiency is working against her.

Fat: Eat Some, Want Some More

As far as Susan's body is concerned, she has just survived a famine, which means that her fat instinct is going to insist that she eat as many calories as she can to buttress herself against the next famine. In its effort to protect itself from the next food shortage (or diet, as Susan would call it), Susan's fat instinct drives her to eat as much fat as she can get down before she is satisfied. In fact, if a meal is rich in fat, we eat much more than we would if the meal was composed chiefly of plant foods. The moment we start to eat a high-fat meal, the fat instinct is triggered, causing us to overeat. If we are hungry when we sit down to a high-fat meal, the fat instinct will cause us to gorge as a way of accumulating enough extra calories to protect our bodies against the next famine.

This phenomenon has been well documented. Cornell researcher Dr. Lauren Lissner compared the number of calories it took to satisfy people on three different diets, each one composed of different amounts of fat. Diet A was low in fat; diet B moderately high in fat; and diet C high in fat. Because all the excess fat was hidden in diets B and C, all three diets appeared essentially the same and all three were rated equally palatable. The study had only two rules: People should eat when hungry, and eat until they felt full. Volunteers were divided into three groups; each group followed each of the three diets for two weeks, after which Dr. Lissner counted the calories it took to satisfy each group on their respective diets. The results were impressive: Dr. Lissner found that people on the high-fat diet ate 658 calories a day more than those on the lower-fat regimens! They weren't satisfied and didn't feel full until they got those 650 additional calories. At that rate, these people will gain about one pound of body fat every five days! In fact, the subjects in the study on the high-fat diet did gain weight and those on the low-fat diet lost weight. Dr. Lissner concluded that the more fat in the diet, the more calories it takes to create satiety.

Cornell researchers did another study to see if the results would be replicated. This time, the volunteers were followed over an eleven-week period. The results were basically the same. As before, those who ate the low-fat diet ate fewer calories and lost weight.

We saw a variation on this theme in the Holt study reported in chapter 1. Holt showed that high-fat foods provide low satiety, which means you have to eat more of these foods in order to feel full. Since high-fat foods have more calories ounce for ounce than most plant foods, they're going to add fat to your body. As if this were not enough, Holt also showed that the consumption of high-fat foods at one meal caused people to eat more calories at their next meal. In other words, the fat instinct triggers a vicious cycle of low satiety and overeating.

High-fat foods increase your weight in three ways:

1. Fat is the most concentrated sources of calories.

2. They increase the likelihood that you will eat more calories at any given meal because they trigger the fat instinct, which encourages you to overeat.

3. They increase the likelihood of overeating at your *next* meal, again because they trigger the fat instinct.

Once the fat instinct is triggered, overeating is an instinctual response that most people cannot control over the long run, no matter how disciplined they may be. This is why people who eat high-fat meals not only eat a lot of calories per sitting, but also feel compelled to eat more fat throughout the day. This is happening to the vast majority of Americans, no matter what their weight. And it's precisely why overweight people—who clearly do not need any more calories—continue to overeat.

MISPLACED BLAME

The minute Susan started regaining her weight, she started to criticize herself relentlessly. Within weeks of stopping her diet, Susan had regained much of the weight she had lost during months of struggle, which made her feel like a complete failure. Susan didn't realize it, but she was not the one to blame for her portion-control diet's failure to help her lose weight and keep it off. The main problem for people who try to lose weight through calorie-restrictive diets is that they require you to be hungry. And chronic hunger is a major trigger of the fat instinct. Because we tend to blame ourselves for failing to meet our weight-loss goals, we don't realize where the real problem lies. Trying to avoid eating in the face of a growing hunger is like trying to stop breathing.

HIGH-PROTEIN DIETS: SHOCK TREATMENT FOR YOUR METABOLISM

Susan is nothing if not relentless. She is a good example of the health instinct in action. The health instinct is the innate desire we all have to be strong, lean of body, and physically fit. The health instinct pushes us to realize our potential in every area of life. Unfortunately, it offers very little guidance on how to achieve our goal of good health. We can very easily find ourselves wandering in the labyrinth of misinformation, which is pretty much what happened to Susan.

Soon she had found another best-selling book that argued for a high-protein, low-carbohydrate diet. The diet made the most appealing of promises: First, Susan could eat foods she had already been eating, such as meat and cheese; second, she would lose weight; and third, she'd never go hungry. It sounded like the perfect diet! All she had to do was avoid carbohydrates. That was the key to the entire program. And indeed, when carbohydrates are severely restricted, the body responds as if it is in famine, which causes a series of chemical changes that result in a suppression of appetite and weight loss. Of course, that's not all that happens, but here's how such diets work.

During normal times when food is available, the body burns a fuel mix that is composed of fat and sugar. That's okay for the body, but not the brain. The brain prefers to burn sugar as its fuel, which it gets from carbohydrate consumption. When a person experiences famine, and carbohydrates are no longer available, the body will burn its sugar reserves, which are stored primarily in your liver and muscles as glycogen. Once those limited reserves are gone, there are only two fuels left: fat, which is stored in the tissues, and protein, which makes up your muscles and other tissues. The brain cannot burn fat directly, so the liver is forced to convert protein into sugar, or glucose, in a process called *gluconeogenesis*. The problem is that during famine, the primary source of protein is your muscles. If you use your muscles as fuel, you'll soon find yourself lacking the strength to hunt for food. It's kind of like burning the wood frame of your house to keep warm. Eventually, the process becomes self-defeating.

The body, in its wisdom, realizes that this is the short road to death. Consequently, after a couple of days of burning protein, the liver performs a wondrous act of chemical ingenuity and converts some of the body's stored fat into *ketones*, which are chemical substances that the brain can use for fuel instead of glucose. Now the body is utilizing its fatty acids, which are being drained from its fat cells, and converting them to ketones so that the brain can survive. The resulting condition, called *ketosis*, is an emergency measure to preserve the body's muscles and vital organs so that people can go on searching for food when they are starving.

Ketosis also causes some suppression of appetite, which is another of the body's remarkable responses to famine: it keeps you from thinking about food, even while you search for it. Ketosis will endure as long as you go without carbohydrates, and as long as you have fat stored in your tissues. The minute you eat a carbohydrate-rich food, however, your body recognizes the presence of its preferred fuel and the liver stops producing ketones. At that point, you are out of ketosis and out of "famine." And, naturally, your fat instinct will drive you to gorge on all the food you can get your hands on.

The only thing you have to do to drive your body into ketosis is to deprive it of carbohydrates for a few days, which is exactly what the architects of the high-protein diets do, and exactly what Susan experienced when she started such a diet.

During the first few days on her diet, Susan's body immediately fell back on its glycogen reserves, the last vestiges of sugar she had stored in her muscles and liver. Glycogen is tied up with the body's water reserves, so the burning of these glycogen stores caused an immediate loss of water, which accounted for much of the weight loss Susan experienced in the first few days of her diet. This was the fast, easy weight loss that is often associated with high-protein diets. Once the body shifted into ketosis and started burning fat, two things happened: First, Susan's appetite was suppressed—a person in ketosis can get by on 600 to 800 calories a day. Second, she lost even more weight. At this point, the weight loss occurred at a slower rate than it did initially, but Susan was still thrilled. Finally, she was losing weight without hunger. Her stomach wasn't constantly nagging her to eat as it had when she was on the portion-control programs; she had no symptoms of the famine response; and she wasn't craving any food. The irony is that at 600 to 800 calories per day, Susan was starving. She just didn't know it.

THE DANGERS OF KETOSIS

In the short run, Susan's high-protein diet was doing all that its proponents had promised it would do, but at what cost? If we look a little closer at what Susan was eating, we can see that she may have been trading one set of problems for another—a set of problems that could be far more severe than overweight. In order to throw her body into ketosis and bring about weight loss, Susan had to severely restrict carbohydrate-rich foods. Of the three macronutrients—carbohydrates, protein, and fat—Susan was eating predominantly protein and fat.

Abundant scientific evidence has shown that a diet rich in fat is linked to numerous life-threatening diseases, including heart disease, adult-onset diabetes, high blood pressure, obesity, and many forms of cancer. Every major scientific health organization, from the National Cancer Institute to the American Heart Association, has urged Americans to reduce fat.

Such recommendations have had little impact on the Pied Pipers of high protein, however. Take a look at some of the recipes found in the best-selling book, *Protein Power*, by Michael R. Eades, M.D., and Mary Dan Eades, M.D. (Bantam, 1996), which includes the recipe for "Finnish Meat Loaf," described as a "typical Finnish meat loaf . . . traditionally wrapped with sour cream pastry and taken along on cross-country skiing picnics. It's delicious either hot or cold and should be served with a big dollop of sour cream." The recipe calls for 4 tablespoons of butter, 3 pounds of ground meat (which includes pork, ham, and veal), 1 cup of grated Gruyère cheese, and ½ cup of heavy cream.

It's worth noting that Finland has among the highest cholesterol levels per capita and, not surprisingly, one of the highest rates of heart disease of any nation on earth. It makes you wonder how many poor Finns, happily sliding through the woods on their cross-country skis, suddenly had fatal heart attacks after eating their famous meat loaf with that "big dollop of sour cream." Other recipes in the book include Veal Scalloppini with Ricotta and Swiss Chard; Spinach, Avocado, Bacon, and Goat Cheese; Tex-Mex Cheese Flan with Chunky Salsa; Butterflied Pork Chops; Warm Brie with Chutney and Almonds . . . I could go on, but you get the picture. The amount of animal fat in these recipes is dangerous, even potentially lethal.

However, fat is not the only macronutrient that people should be concerned about when adopting a high-protein diet. Such diets rely heavily upon animal proteins, which studies suggest may independently raise your risk of disease. Among the illnesses that excess animal proteins may contribute to are certain types of cancer, gout, kidney disease, and osteoporosis.

When the National Cancer Institute and the American Heart Association urge Americans to reduce fat, they also are implicitly urging people to reduce animal protein, because protein-rich foods are tremendous sources of fat and cholesterol. There's a good scientific reason for making such a recommendation. When scientists look around the world to find those people who experience low rates of the major degenerative diseases, they find a consistent pattern: The people who subsist on diets low in fat and moderately low in protein—especially animal proteins—have the lowest rates of heart disease, cancer, high blood pressure, adult-onset diabetes, and other major illnesses.

The Pritikin diet provides optimal amounts of protein. In fact, our diet contains about the same amount of protein as the typical American diet. We do include animal proteins, but we rely most heavily on plant proteins, which are the greatest sources of antioxidants, phytochemicals, and other immune-boosting and cancer-protecting compounds. They are also rich in fiber. Consequently, when you eat the protein in the Pritikin diet, you also get a wide array of other health-promoters.

As I have already shown, animal foods are low in these immune-boosting chemicals and devoid of fiber. Low-fiber diets are associated with a host of digestive disorders, including constipation, diverticulosis, hemorrhoids, and colon cancer.

Susan was aware of these long-term health concerns and such knowledge threw her into conflict over her high-protein diet. She enjoyed losing the weight, but she knew that she was consuming a diet that might be a formula for disease. The experience was all too reminiscent of her years in college when she smoked cigarettes to dampen her appetite and lose weight. She knew she was compromising her health and increasing the likelihood that she would get seriously ill, if not immediately then perhaps years down the road.

Like many people who are seduced by the promises of high-protein diets, Susan was gambling that she could use the diet for its only short-term benefit—weight loss—and then dump it before she suffered any long-term consequences. What she didn't realize is that there are short-term consequences to such regimens as well.

Even in the short-run, high-protein diets can increase the likelihood of suffering from gout, kidney stones, bone-weakening calcium loss, and orthostatic hypotension, which decreases blood flow to the brain, especially in the elderly, and is oftentimes accompanied by dizziness and fainting. In addition, because high-protein diets provide relatively small amounts of carbohydrates, adherents often lack the energy to exercise. With less exercise, dieters have a tendency to lose more muscle mass while on high-protein diets. As I will show, maintaining muscle mass is crucial to long-term weight loss. Finally, all those fatty animal foods train the palate to prefer a rich fatty diet, which makes switching to a low-fat, health-promoting program exceedingly difficult.

Don't Go Near the Bread; It'll Kill the Diet!

Soon, Susan found herself craving the very food she was told to stay away from: carbohydrates. Evolution has designed the human body to eat a diet made up predominantly of plant foods rich in carbohydrates. All of our urgent energy needs—our ability to react quickly to a stimulus—depend on carbohydrates in the blood, liver, and muscles. Unfortunately, on a high-protein ketotic diet, those carbohydrate stores just aren't there.

Not surprisingly, Susan found that after a few weeks on her high-protein diet she was craving cakes, rolls, bread, and pastries. And then one day, her cravings got the best of her and she ate a roll. The minute she ate a carbohydrate-rich food, several metabolic reactions occurred. Suddenly, Susan's body could burn carbohydrates, its preferred fuel, instead of ketones. "I'm out of ketosis," the brain shouts. "I'm no longer starving!" When the body and brain stop burning ketones, the appetite-suppressing effects of the ketones disappear. Susan had been getting by on 600 to 800 calories a day. Instantly, she realizes that she is famished. Not only that, but the foods she wants the most are pastries, rolls, breads, ice cream, and sweets.

Very often, people coming off a high-protein diet binge on processed carbohydrates that contain both fat and sugar: doughnuts, Danish, ice cream, and cakes. In fact, they crave all sources of carbohydrates, including brown rice, vegetables, and fruits, but they want the most concentrated sources of carbohydrates, which are processed foods and foods rich in sugar.

Once a person who has been starving for carbohydrates on a high-protein diet starts to eat rich foods, most of the fat contained in those foods is quickly stored in the tissues: in other words, Susan started gaining weight again. Once again, biology had defeated her willpower.

Carbohydrate consumption is the undoing of the ketotic dietary approach, because as soon as you eat a carbohydrate-rich food, your body is driven to gorge. Once you've done that, you're out of ketosis and your long-suppressed appetite returns with a vengeance.

HYBRID DIETS

A few high-protein diets try to get around the body's natural craving for carbohydrates by allowing small amounts of them. Proponents of these diets realize that carbohydrate craving is often the undoing of the high-protein regimen. However, the minute you include more than one or two ounces of carbohydrates in a high-protein, high-fat diet, you've got to limit the size of the portions you eat. By including carbohydrates, you will prevent significant ketosis, which in turn will also prevent appetite suppression. You're going to feel how hungry you are, which means that you will overeat and gain weight.

The only way around this problem is to strictly limit the size of your meals, or invoke portion control, which will reduce your calorie consumption. So now you're really on a high-protein, portion-control diet. You have to use portion control because of the high-fat content of the diet, which provides an abundance of calories. Of course, the minute you start limiting the size of your meals, you're going to be hungry. And being hungry will trigger your fat instinct. At that point, it's only a matter of time before you give in to your craving.

THE COST OF STARVATION IS HIGH

Both portion-control and high-protein diets cause their own kinds of starvation, resulting in calorie and nutrient deficits. Such losses cause you to lose both fat and muscle tissue. Muscle is the worst type of tissue to lose for anyone who wants to lose weight, because it is highly active and continually burning fat. If your body has a proportionately high degree of muscle tissue, you'll burn more calories throughout the day. So one of the keys to weight loss is to protect muscle mass while you reduce calories. But on a high-protein or portion-control diet, you don't have the energy to exercise, which means you will lose muscle as you lose fat.

High-carbohydrate diets protect muscles better than other weight-loss programs. But even more, high-carbohydrate diets give you the energy to exercise while you are losing weight, which means you can protect your muscle mass, and even increase it, while you burn fat. In fact, the only diet that helps you lose weight without hunger and gives you plenty of energy to exercise is a high-carbohydrate, low-fat diet.

BILL'S STORY

Bill Hughes was just thirty-five years old in 1986, but he already suffered with high blood pressure and weighed 283 pounds. A self-proclaimed type-A personality and a hard-driving businessman, Bill woke up one day, looked in the mirror, and realized that he fit the profile for a heart attack victim perfectly. "I was killing myself," he said.

Bill was so overweight, his chest and stomach so distended, that he couldn't bend over in most small chairs to tie his shoes. Bill's two children were both young—one two years old and the other six months—when he realized he had to do something to help himself survive long enough to watch his kids grow up. "Just carrying my young sons up the stairs made me huff and puff. . . . Here I was, only thirty-five years old. . . . I thought, My God, am I going to be around for these little boys?"

In February 1987 he began the Pritikin Program and in a matter of a few months had lost forty pounds. Nine months later, he lost eighty pounds and has kept it off ever since. In 1996 Bill was the CEO of a multistate waste equipment manufacturing company, a community leader, a husband, and a father. He's also in the best shape of his life.

"I'm doing things at forty-five that at age thirty-five I never would have thought of doing," he said. His passion is serious mountain climbing: Mont Blanc on the French-Italian border, Mount Rainier in Washington State; Chimborazo in Ecuador; Orizaba in Mexico; Lenin Peak in Kyrgyzstan; Mount Elbrus, Russia. You have to be in shape to climb these mountains, but Bill is up to it.

"Every extra pound you try to carry up a mountain, whether it's in your backpack or on your stomach, is an absolute killer," says Bill. "The fitter you are, the better, the more exhilarating the experience."

Proponents of portion-control and ketotic weight-loss programs are attempting to sell us diets that will satisfy both our fat instincts and our desire to be slim and healthy. Unfortunately, the two are incompatible. Still, you can't blame yourself for wanting to try them. But as we all eventually find out, there are no simple solutions. Programs that by their very nature trigger the fat instinct will set you up for failure. Those who follow that path eventually get tired and frustrated with diets. Many choose to try one of the weight-reducing drugs; others opt for some form of surgery. Eventually, these high-fat, high-protein diets may cause serious disease. No wonder so many people have chosen to give up the whole business of trying to reestablish their health and optimal weight and have taken up the "pleasure revenge," as Faith Popcorn so aptly terms such behavior. People are angry because they have made sacrifices, they've worked hard for better health and optimal weight, and yet they are still gaining weight. Frankly, I don't blame them one bit. As long as people do not know how to overcome their fat instincts, there is no diet out there that can succeed, which means, sadly, that health is beyond the reach of most of us. The pleasure revenge is the ultimate victory of the fat instinct.

WEIGHT LOSS
WITHOUT HUNGER

Susan realized after she gave birth that she had to do something extraordinary to lose weight. At first, she didn't know what she could do. She'd tried every kind of diet imaginable, or so she thought. Susan lives in Santa Monica, California, not far from our center, but she never considered the Pritikin diet because she had the false idea that our program focuses only on overcoming serious illnesses, such as heart disease. "I thought that Pritikin is for people who are seriously ill, not overweight," Susan recalled. "The only thing I was sick of was being fat."

Another reason why Susan believed that we couldn't help her with her weight was that she knew our diet is composed of a lot of carbohydrates, which she had read are terrible for weight loss. One book said that carbohydrates are loaded with calories, which turn into fat. Another said that carbohydrates drive up insulin levels, which prevent you from burning fat that's already stored on your body.

The diets Susan had been on in the past required her to limit the size of her meals, which meant that she was hungry most of the time. When she dropped the portion-control diets, she adopted high-protein regimens. These diets, in fact, gave her the biggest initial weight loss, but like the portion-control programs, they were too restrictive to follow for very long. Susan was also concerned that a diet based mainly on meat and eggs would increase her risk of heart disease and cancer. Soon after adopting the program, she inexplicably started eating everything in sight and regained her weight.

Susan would have continued adopting new diets—and surely would have continued failing at them—were it not for a serendipitous event that turned her in a new direction. Susan had a friend who attended the Pritikin P.M. Program, which is a nonresident course designed to allow local people to attend the lectures, eat the food, and participate in our exercise program at the center during the evenings. As it happened, Susan bumped into her friend, who had lost a significant amount of weight on our program and was having no trouble keeping the weight off.

"What happened to you?" Susan asked her friend after she hadn't seen her in quite some time. "You look wonderful!" Susan admits today that she was almost in awe of the transformation her friend had undergone. Not only was she slim and fit, but she looked younger. Susan's friend explained that she had attended the Longevity Center in the evenings and had lost more than fifty pounds. The next day, Susan was at the counter of the Longevity Center signing up for the P.M. Program. The following Monday night, she attended my workshop on the fat instinct, and for the first time understood why a high-carbohydrate diet caused weight loss without ever making you go hungry. Susan also understood why so many diets had failed her, and would keep on failing her until she either gave up on diets or learned to outsmart her fat instinct.

PLANTS: LOW-CALORIE, HIGH-FIBER FOODS THAT FILL YOU UP

Contrary to some erroneous but widely held notions, plant foods are the basis for effective weight loss. The reason is simple: Plant foods have the fewest calories. When you consider the calorie content of any food, it's helpful to look at the food from the standpoint of "calorie-density" or "calorie-concentration," which means the number of calories packed into a given amount of that food. Calories is another word for the amount of potential fuel that can be found in a food product. You can get calories from carbohydrates or fat, but there's a big difference between how many calories are concentrated in a gram of carbohydrate versus a gram of fat. As I mentioned in chapter 1, a gram of carbohydrate has 4 calories, while a gram of fat contains 9 calories. Most plant foods contain a rich supply of fiber and water, and modest amounts of protein. The vast majority of plant foods contain very little fat, which means they are calorically "sparse" or "light." Animal foods are "calorically dense," because they contain no fiber, but significant amounts of fat.

In essence, plant foods are packaged water; the water is held within the plant by fiber. Together, the fiber and the water make plant foods bulky. Since water contains no calories, and fiber only minute amounts, plant foods fill you up without adding weight to your body. Let's compare some plant foods with high-protein, high-fat animal foods to see what the calorie differences are.

A large $3^{1}/_{2}$-ounce tomato contains 21 calories. Three and a half ounces of lean ground beef contains 300 calories. The tomato contains less than a tenth of the calories as the same size portion of red meat.

The calorie content of a tomato is typical of vegetables. Three and a half ounces of butternut squash has 45 calories. The same size serving of an onion has 38 calories, and of collard greens, 19 calories. All of these vegetables have negligible amounts of fat and plenty of fiber.

Among the most calorically concentrated vegetables is a potato. A $3^{1}/_{2}$-ounce baked potato has about 109 calories. The same size serving of sweet potato has about 105 calories. When you examine the calorie content of various cuts of beef, all $3^{1}/_{2}$-ounce servings, you get a range of about 219 calories (for the arm) to about 300 calories for short ribs. Your average $3^{1}/_{2}$-ounce sirloin steak has anywhere from 200 to 237 calories. And after all the peripheral fat has been trimmed away, that steak still derives more than 40 percent of its calories from fat.

Three-and-a-half ounces of meat is only about the size of a deck of cards. Most people I know eat at least an 8- to 12-ounce piece of meat when they sit down to a meal. Because you need more of a high-fat food to create satiety, you're going to feel cheated if you eat only a small piece of beef, or lamb, or pork; that small piece of meat will not fill you up. That means, of course, that $3^{1}/_{2}$ ounces of meat is not a good yardstick for most people measuring the calorie content of what they actually eat. As you increase the size of the portion, you also increase the calorie content. Moreover, meat will trigger your fat instinct and almost guarantee that you will eat more calories—either in the form of more meat and fat, or from other foods at the same meal, such as a baked potato with sour cream.

But you'd be surprised how satisfying a small piece of meat can be when used as part of a beef stew or fish or chicken soup, which is exactly how we use meat, fish, and chicken in our Pritikin recipes. We add lots of vegetables and spices to these dishes, making them hearty, filling, and delicious. When used in this way, you get the palatability of the meat and the satiety of the vegetables.

There's no comparison between the calorie content of a plant-based meal versus the calorie content of your average American meal. In addition, their capacities to create satiety are vastly different. The majority of plant foods are so low in calories that you can eat great volumes of them and still only get 500 calories. Because plants fill you up on relatively few calories, it's tough to eat more than two small sweet potatoes at a single meal; however, even if you ate three of them, you're not going to get many calories (315) and you're going to be stuffed. The sheer mass of food that you are eating in a plant-based meal will stretch your stomach receptors so that your brain will be telling you "I'm full," even though you've just eaten a low-calorie meal. On the other hand, you can sit down to a big fast-food meal that includes a double-cheeseburger, a milk shake, and fries, and eat 1,200-plus calories without blinking an eye.

The point here is that most unprocessed plant foods are naturally low in calories, while high-protein, high-fat foods are high in calories.

A typical American high-fat diet has high calorie-concentration at every meal. That's why you've got to limit the size of your meals, because the more fat you take in, the more weight you're going to gain. But the consequences of portion control are chronic hunger, a slowed metabolic rate, and obsession with food.

On the Pritikin Program, you can eat as much food as you want, whenever you want. You're still going to lose weight, because the number of calories you eat will be less than what your body burns as fuel each day. People on our program lose weight gradually and safely, and they never go hungry.

CANCER FIGHTERS AND IMMUNE BOOSTERS

When I think about why people should eat plant foods, I'm reminded of John Dillinger's reply to the question, Why do you rob banks, Mr. Dillinger? "Because that's where the money is."

Why should we eat plant foods? Because that's where the nutrition is.

When nutritionists talk about food, they usually talk about two groups of nutrients: the big nutrients, also called *macronutrients*, which are fat, protein, and carbohydrates, and the little ones, called *micro-*

SOURCES OF MACRONUTRIENTS		
Sources of Fat	*Sources of Protein*	*Sources of Carbohydrates*
All red meats, including all forms of beef, pork, ham	All red meats	Whole grains, such as brown rice, millet, corn, oats, wheat, barley
All whole dairy products, including whole milk, cheeses, sour cream, whipped cream	Chicken	Green and leafy vegetables, such as collard, kale, mustard greens, broccoli, brussels sprouts, lettuce, cabbage
	Eggs	
	Dairy foods	
	Fish	
	Plants: All grains, vegetables, beans, nuts, seeds (these plant foods contain moderate and healthful amounts of protein)	
Eggs that include the yolks		Root vegetables, such as carrots, parsnips, turnips, ginger
Chicken, especially the dark meat and the skin		Tubers, such as potatoes, sweet potatoes, yams, rutabaga
Plant foods: Avocados, olives, seeds, nuts		Red and yellow vegetables, such as tomatoes, squash
		Fruit
		Milk (lactose, a milk sugar, is a source of carbohydrates)

nutrients, which include vitamins, and minerals. In addition to these two categories, there is a third group called *phytochemicals,* which include literally hundreds of newly discovered chemicals that boost your immune system and help you fight cancer.

Protein and fat are found mostly in animal foods, while carbohydrates are found primarily in plant foods, such as grains, beans, vegetables, and fruits. Some plant foods have moderate amounts of protein; others have small amounts. Most plant foods are extremely low in fat, with a few exceptions, namely olives, avocados, nuts, and seeds. There are some fairly low-fat animal foods, such as skim milk, most fish, and the white meat of chicken (without the skin), but most animal foods contain significant amounts of fat and all contain cholesterol. Thus, most high-protein, low-carbohydrate foods are animal foods, most of which are high in fat; the vast majority of high-carbohydrate, moderate-protein foods are plant foods, most of which are low in fat.

Each of the three macronutrients has its own specific role to play in the body. Dietary fat is used by the body as a source of fuel; it's also needed in small amounts to absorb and help transport the fat-soluble vitamins, A, D, E, and K in the body. Protein is used by the body for cell growth, replacement, and repair. Carbohydrates are the body's source of fuel for all urgent energy needs. They are converted in the body into glucose, or blood sugar, which is then used by cells as fuel.

So when your diet is composed mostly of plant foods, you will be getting a lot of carbohydrates, adequate amounts of protein, and very little fat. You'll also be getting lots of fiber. Only plant foods have fiber. Fiber is essential to healthy digestion and the elimination of many harmful cellular by-products, including cancer-promoting estrogens.

Sources of Micronutrients

In addition to providing carbohydrates, plant foods are also the richest sources of most micronutrients, such as vitamins, minerals, and many cancer-fighting and immune-boosting substances. The only exceptions are vitamins B_{12} and D, which I discussed in chapter 2.

Some of the most exciting research in health and nutrition science concerns plant chemicals, also referred to as phytochemicals. Substances that scientists call antioxidants, phytochemicals, indoles, bioflavonoids, and carotenoids appear to boost our immune systems and help to protect us against cancer and heart disease. Science is demonstrating that many of these micronutrients protect DNA from mutating and triggering malignancies; others promote the cancer-fighting mechanisms in cells; and still others boost the body's ability to ward off all kinds of diseases that threaten us daily, including heart disease and cataracts.

It's worth noting that when these nutrients are isolated and put in pill form, they do not necessarily have the same beneficial effects as when you get them from your food. Recent large-scale experiments have indicated that high-dose supplements of beta carotene may increase a smoker's risk of getting cancer. However, when you get beta carotene and other antioxidants from food, they are associated with lower rates of cancer.

All of these health-promoting substances are found in plants. Animal foods are very good sources of some individual micronutrients, such as iron or calcium, but they contain few or no antioxidants, carotenoids, and many other essential micronutrients.

SOURCES OF BETA CAROTENE

There is no established Recommended Daily Amount (RDA) for beta carotene, but scientists recommend that people get between 10 and 30 milligrams (mg) per day.

Food Animal	Serving Size	Amount (mg)	% Daily Requirement
Red meat	N/A	0	0
Dairy foods (milk and cheese)	N/A	0	0
Eggs	N/A	0	0
Fish	N/A	0	0
Vegetables			
Brussels sprouts	1/2 cup	3.4	11
Carrots	1 medium	12.2	41
Kale	1/2 cup	8.2	27
Mustard greens	1/2 cup	7.3	24
Spinach	1/2 cup	4.4	15
Squash	1/2 cup	16.1	54
Sweet Potato	1 medium	2.9	10

SOURCES OF BETA CAROTENE, *Continued*

Fruit

Apricots	3 medium	1.7	6
Cantaloupe	½ medium	5.2	17
Mango	1 medium	4.8	16

SOURCES OF VITAMIN C

Animal	Serving Size	Amount (mg)	% Daily Requirement (60 mg)
Red meat	N/A	0	0
Dairy foods	N/A	0	0
Eggs	N/A	0	0
Fish	N/A	0	0
Vegetables			
Broccoli	½ cup	49	82
Cabbage	½ cup	17	28
Cauliflower	½ cup	34	57
Chili pepper	½ cup	109	182
Collard greens	½ cup	9	15
Green bell pepper	1 medium	95	158
Kale	½ cup	51	85
Peas (canned)	½ cup	12	20
Peas (fresh)	½ cup	38	63
Potato (baked)	1 medium	26	43
Sauerkraut	½ cup	17	28
Winter squash	½ cup	10	17
Fruit			
Cantaloupe	½ medium	113	188
Grapefruit	½ medium	41	68
Oranges	1 medium	70	117
Papaya	1 medium	188	313
Strawberries	1 cup	85	142

SOURCES OF VITAMIN E

Animal	Serving Size	Amount (mg)	% Daily Requirement (10 mg)
Red meat	N/A	0	0
Dairy foods	N/A	0	0
Eggs	N/A	0	0
Fish			
Cod	3 oz.	0.8	8
Mackerel	3 oz.	1.5	15
Salmon (broiled or canned)	3 oz.	1.6–1.8	16–18
Shrimp (broiled)	3 oz.	0.6–3.5	6–35
Grains/Breads			
Brown rice	1/2 cup	1.2	12
Seven-grain bread	1 slice	0.3	3
Wheat bread	1 slice	0.2	2
White bread	1 slice	0.3	3
White rice	1/2 cup	0.4	4
Wild rice	1/2 cup	1.8	18
Seeds and Nuts			
Almonds	1 oz.	5.0	50
Peanuts	1 oz.	3.1	31
Sunflower seeds	1 oz.	14.8	148
Vegetables			
Asparagus	1/2 cup	1.8	18
Beets	1/2 cup	2.0	20
Kidney beans	1/2 cup	4.4	44
Pinto or lima beans	1/2 cup	4.1	41
Spinach	1/2 cup	1.9	19
Sweet potato	1 medium	5.5	55
Fruit			
Apple	1 medium	0.4	4
Mango	1 medium	2.7	27
Pear	1 medium	1.3	13

If you want to eat a diet that will help to prevent cancer, heart disease, and other degenerative illnesses, you've got to eat lots of plant foods, such as whole grains, fresh vegetables, beans, and fruit, which means you've got to eat carbohydrates.

BUT CARBOHYDRATES ARE SUPPOSED TO CAUSE WEIGHT GAIN

But wait a minute, you may be saying. What about the fact that some people eat carbohydrates and gain weight? You're absolutely right. Some people do eat carbohydrates and gain weight, because not all carbohydrate foods are the same. In fact, there is a big difference between a bowl of oatmeal, or carrots, or fruit, for example, and a pastry, or a doughnut, or even a slice of white bread. These foods have vastly different effects on your appetite and weight, and—as we will see in the next chapter—on your fat instinct.

DAN'S STORY

Dan Jones (a pseudonym) entered politics when he was in his twenties and eventually became his state's speaker of the house and lieutenant governor. A dozen years later, he went into business and real estate, where he prospered beyond his wildest dreams. In 1994, when he was fifty-five years old, Dan was forty pounds overweight, and he didn't like it. "I made up my mind that I wanted to weigh less than I did when I was in high school."

Being on a weight-loss program was not going to be easy, however. Dan traveled all over the world; he had a lot of social engagements that required that he eat in restaurants and, afterward, drink with prospective clients. "My diet was red meat, alcohol, and caffeine," he recalled. "I did everything you shouldn't be doing to your system." Still, he carried his 245 pounds well. "Physically, I didn't really have to lose the weight. At six-four, I'm a large frame, so I could hide forty pounds and not look too bad."

The only problem was that he didn't feel well. "I knew that I had to get my life under control. It was time I changed my lifestyle."

Dan found the Pritikin Program, lost forty pounds in a few months, and shrank his waist size from 42 inches to 37. Eighteen months later, when we checked with him again, he was still 205 pounds, as tall and lean as he had been in high school.

Despite his schedule and his travels, he has no trouble remaining on the program. He uses the exercise facilities at hotels when he's on the road; orders vegetarian meals in advance on airplanes ("I've discovered that the low-fat meals on airplanes are not as good as the vegetarian meals"); and has no trouble ordering healthfully in restaurants. At home, it's easy to maintain both the program and his pattern of frequent eating.

"I'm much better off with four or five smaller meals throughout the day, rather than . . . one big blow-out at the end of the day. I don't like to go to major meals hungry."

For breakfast, Dan has oatmeal or cereal and fruit. A couple of hours later, he eats a cup of soup or some vegetables; at lunchtime, pasta ("there are good pasta places near my office") and a vegetable plate, or he goes to a deli and has half of a turkey breast sandwich and a cup of soup. Midafternoon, he eats another snack ("even if it's just pretzels"). At dinner, he and his wife, Marie, go out to a local restaurant, usually vegetarian, Italian, Mexican, or Asian. And at night, he has any one of several healthful snacks.

"What's wonderful about Pritikin, I think, is that anyone can do it. At first, of course, it takes some fortitude, but there isn't anyone who can't get healthier by following this lifestyle."

5

CARBOHYDRATES: THE REAL STORY

A lot has been written recently about carbohydrates, most of it critical and confusing, especially when it comes to weight loss. As I travel around the country lecturing about diet and health, I find that no other food creates more bewilderment among people today. Mention the word carbohydrate and right away people think of sugar or bread. "Don't both cause weight gain?" people ask me. "Yes, they can" I tell them. People nod their heads with recognition. "We should stay away from carbohydrates in order to lose weight," someone in the audience will say.

"Actually, you should eat carbohydrate-rich foods if you want to lose weight and never be hungry," I tell my listeners. Now people are really baffled. "But I thought you said that carbohydrate foods cause weight gain."

"Some do and some don't," I say. "Did you know that brown rice, apples, pasta, bread, and doughnuts are all carbohydrate-rich foods, but some of these foods have very different effects on your weight than others? Some of these foods are ideal for losing weight, while others will add fat to your body even before you have finished eating them."

Carbohydrates are not just sugary foods or bread products. In fact, there's a whole world of foods that fall under the general rubric of carbohydrates. And they can be as different from each other as carrots and candy canes.

THE REAL THING AND THE IMPOSTORS

Carbohydrates occur in two forms: complex carbohydrates and simple sugars. Complex carbohydrates are long chains of sugar molecules, all wrapped in fiber and water. You eat them every time you eat a whole grain, vegetable, or fruit. Simple sugars appear as individual sugar molecules, or as pairs of sugar molecules. In nature, they turn up most commonly in fruit, where they are still wrapped in fiber and water.

When you eat a whole grain, bean, vegetable, or fruit, your intestinal tract has to work hard to break down the plant and remove the individual sugars from the fiber and the complex chain within which the sugars are held. You can visualize this chain of sugars as a train of boxcars, with each boxcar representing an individual sugar unit. Each boxcar has to be broken off and absorbed by your small intestine, which allows the sugars to enter your bloodstream in a slow, methodical manner. Once inside your bloodstream, these sugars can be used as fuel or stored in the liver or muscle as glycogen.

The sugars are trapped inside the fiber, and the process of extracting them from the fiber is laborious. Humans have a long digestive tract because your intestines need to work on carbohydrates for a long time in order to free the sugars from them. Our entire digestive process was created to release the plant's sugars from the fiber so that we could use them as energy.

This long and involved digestive process causes sugar to drip into your bloodstream at a rate of a few calories per minute. This means that the sugars are slowly absorbed into your bloodstream. It can take hours to fully digest a meal of grains, beans, vegetables, or fruit. Because the rate of absorption is so slow, the process gives you a steady stream of energy and vitality between meals. This may be why people who eat whole grains, fresh vegetables, beans, and fruit have long-lasting energy: the foods themselves are rich in carbohydrates, and these carbohydrates provide a steady supply of sugars to the body over a long period of time.

Two important points to remember about the carbohydrates found in natural plant foods are, in general, that (1) they are low in calories and (2) their calories are slowly absorbed over many hours of digestion.

As long as the sugars are in plants, it doesn't matter if they are complex carbohydrates or simple sugars: the body still has to work hard to get those calories out of the fiber, and that takes time.

Whenever I mention the word sugar in one of my talks, a certain percentage of my listeners will feel guilty because they love sweet foods, but they think of their preference for sweet taste as a form of weakness. But then I tell them we were all designed by nature to prefer sweet foods. In fact, it's one of the reasons we survived as a species.

The Advantages of a Sweet Tooth

One of the distinguishing features of carbohydrates is that they are sweet. Humans developed a sweet tooth in order to determine that a food was ripe. Sweet flavor meant that a food was safe and ready to be eaten. Many unripe fruits contain toxins that keep animals away until the fruit and its seeds are mature. Once the plant is ready to release its seeds to germinate in the soil, the fruit becomes sweet, enticing people, birds, and other animals to eat the proverbial apple—or pear—and drop its seeds on the ground. Even more important, sweet taste informed ancient humans that the food had reached its maximum nutritional value. Thus, sweetness came to mean a nutritious, safe food that contained calories or energy.

During our entire evolution, plant foods (or carbohydrates) were eaten with minimal processing and virtually no refining. All of that changed with the advent of modern food processing, which turned our natural and healthy desire for sweet-tasting foods against us.

PROCESSING AND REFINING: DESTROYING THE HARVEST

When you look out over a field of golden wheat, or rows of corn or rice, or walk through an apple orchard with its ripe fruit popping out like little gifts glistening in the sunlight, you're looking at plant foods as nature intended them to be eaten. Unfortunately, many of the fruits from our "amber waves of grain" and bucolic orchards go straight from the farm to the food processing plant, where three possible fates await them: they can be *processed* or *refined* or *both*.

When a plant food is processed, it is altered by milling, grinding, pulverizing, sifting, juicing, drying, reheating, dehydrating, reconstituting, or boiling. Food manufacturers can also refine a natural plant food, which strips away most of its fiber and often many nutrients as well. In the strict sense, processing and refining are two different techniques, but for the sake of simplicity, and because so many foods are both processed and refined, I will occasionally refer to both of these techniques when I use the word processing.

Processing and refining can do two things to food: they alter the structure of carbohydrate molecules, making them easier and faster to absorb; and they can separate the fiber and water, leaving behind more concentrated calories.

Usually, the net effect of processing or refining is to turn the processed food into a bigger source of calories than it was in its natural state.

Consider, for example, the processing of corn. Corn is a natural plant food made up of complex carbohydrates, all bound together in water and fiber. Food manufacturers can process the corn and turn it into cornstarch, which means they've taken a large volume of corn and broken it down into a relatively small volume of powdery cornstarch. You probably couldn't eat all the corn it takes to produce a single-handful of cornstarch. Yet, that small amount of cornstarch is loaded with calories. In fact, none of the calories in the original large volume of corn have been lost. They've just been packed into a smaller volume of food by removing the fiber and water.

The processing of apples is another good example. A pound of apples contains about 263 calories; a pound of apple butter, which is a processed and concentrated food made from many apples, contains about 844 calories. Since evolution trained us to select the sweetest food possible—that was always the one with the most nutrition and calories—many of us naturally prefer the apple butter to the apple. But in our modern food supply, the healthier food—and the best one for weight loss—is the apple, which is lower in calories and has more fiber.

Of course, part of food processing often involves adding artificial ingredients and/or fat. The healthful potato is turned into a calorie-dense monster when you process it and add fat. Two big baked potatoes (which amount to a little less than a pound) contain approximately 440 calories. If you process those potatoes and add fat, you can turn that pound of potatoes into a pound of French fries, which contains 1,216 calories. If you process the potato even further and add oil, you can turn that potato into potato chips. One pound of potato chips contains 2,576 calories. Even a pound of sugar has only 1,750 calories.

Not only are you getting lots of calories, but also consuming lots of fat. Many processed foods, especially bakery products, have fat added to them, which means that you will eat lots of extra calories before you are full.

Processed carbohydrates that are not sources of concentrated calories are those that are cooked in water, such as pasta and oatmeal. Pasta and rolled oats have similar effects on your body as unprocessed foods, such as beans, corn, and brown rice. They're low in calorie-concentration. Thus, if you eat whole wheat spaghetti noodles, or even a refined white noodle, with marinara sauce that contains little or no oil, it's unlikely you will gain weight.

A processed food is no longer a natural plant food, because natural plant foods are calorically sparse, while a processed food tends to be calorically dense. In addition, the most highly processed foods tend to have all or most of their fiber and many other nutrients removed.

A processed food that's often thought of as good for weight loss because it is fat-free is dried cereal. Unfortunately, the calories in these foods are so concentrated that they typically contain as much as 1,750 calories per pound, most of which are rapidly absorbed, which means they make it more difficult to lose weight. But let's be clear: we're talking about degrees of influence on your weight. If you're used to eating steak and bacon, a fat-free dried cereal will be a lot better for your weight—and your health—than your previous high-fat choices. Cooked oatmeal, on the other hand, contains about 500 calories per pound, and is slowly absorbed. Also, because it is less processed and less concentrated, it provides greater satiety so you will eat fewer calories. It's clearly the better breakfast choice for anyone interested in weight loss.

MAINLINING CALORIES

In general, the carbohydrates in plant foods are low in calories and slowly absorbed largely because they are all bound up in fiber and water. Processed foods are very different, however. First, they have had their calories concentrated, so that you are often eating a food that is loaded with calories—even though it may be "fat-free." Second, the chemical structure of the food may have been changed, or the calories themselves have been extracted from the fiber, allowing the calories or sugars in the food to be rapidly absorbed into your bloodstream. The sugars in such a processed food flow immediately into your bloodstream, flooding your blood with sugar. By processing and refining the food, the factory has done the job of extracting the sugars from the fiber. It has, in effect, *predigested* your food. Once the food enters your small intestine, its sugars are immediately absorbed.

Thus, when foods are processed, two things usually happen:

1. The water has been removed so that the calories are concentrated.

2. The fiber has been removed and the chemical structure of the food has been disrupted, making the calories rapidly absorbed into the bloodstream. In this way, the food has been predigested in the factory.

What's so terrible about having lots of sugar and calories enter your bloodstream all at once? And what's all this got to do with weight loss?

Let me give you the short version first. The calories from processed food flood your bloodstream and must be burned quickly or stored to maintain health. Ordinarily, you burn a fuel mix of both fat and sugar, but when your blood is overwhelmed by sugars from processed carbo-hydrates, you burn primarily sugar and store most of the fat. Storing extra dietary fat while not burning your body fat means you're gaining weight.

How Insulin Regulates Weight

Eating a processed food causes your bloodstream to be flooded with an abundance of sugar (read calories) all at once. Exceedingly high blood sugar, when maintained over time, is a life-threatening disease called diabetes. Diabetes is associated with a range of side effects, including heart disease, kidney failure, poor circulation, blindness, and gangrene. If high blood sugar levels are allowed to persist, they can cause nerve, eye, kidney, and vascular damage.

The body protects itself against the consequent damage caused by excess sugar in the blood. High levels of sugar signal your pancreas to produce lots of insulin, which is secreted into the bloodstream. Insulin is a hormone that acts like a kind of doorman, allowing sugar to pass from the outside of a cell's wall to the inside, so that your cell can utilize the sugar as fuel or store it as glycogen. When you eat a meal of processed and refined foods, a lot of sugar floods into your bloodstream, which means you need a lot of little doormen to let the sugar pass into your cells. Your pancreas responds by producing a lot of insulin. Immediately, your insulin levels jump up—it's called an insulin spike—so that sugar can be allowed inside the cells.

Your body reacts very aggressively to an insulin spike. The first thing it tries to do with a sudden rush of sugar is to store it safely as blood sugar, in the form of glycogen. Blood sugar is stored in your muscles and your liver; however, the liver's capacity to store glycogen is significantly less than that of the muscles. The muscles of an average woman can store about 1,000 calories; those of an average man, about 1,500 calories. The amount varies depending on the size of your muscles—men tend to have bigger muscles than women—and whether or not you have recently exercised. If you exercised vigorously, the reserves of glycogen in your muscles will be low, which means that you'll have room to store more blood sugar. If you haven't exercised today, then your muscles will be full, which means there will be no room to store the sudden rush of excess sugar.

Let's assume that your liver and muscles are pretty full. What happens to the sugar? Contrary to what many people believe, sugar is rarely converted to fat. The conversion of sugar to fat requires too much energy from the body. The body sees no point in burning lots of energy just to store a little. Also, you can't store sugar in any great quantities in your tissues. Calorie for calorie, stored fat is eight times lighter than stored glycogen or protein. Trees store carbohydrates rather than fat, but humans need a reserve fuel that's light and highly mobile; fat fits the bill perfectly.

When the storage tanks in the liver and muscles are full, the only practical thing your body can do with excess blood sugar is to burn it as fuel. Moreover, because high blood sugar is dangerous, it has to be burned fast; otherwise, you're going to get sick.

Right now, as you read this book, you're probably burning a fuel mix of about 50 percent sugar and 50 percent fat; however, that 50-50 ratio depends on what you have recently eaten. Let's say that before you picked up this book, you ate a pastry, which flooded your blood with sugar. Your body has to burn that blood sugar immediately, which means that your body has to change its fuel mix. It does this by decreasing its fat burning so that it can burn more sugar in the shortest amount of time. Now your fuel mix consists almost entirely of sugar. What happens to the fat that would have been burned? It stays in your tissues, which is exactly what every dieter wants to avoid. Even worse, eating processed food that includes both fat and concentrated carbohydrates forces the storage of the incoming fat so that the sugar can be burned off quickly. Consequently, when you eat pastries, doughnuts, or muffins that contain both fat and sugar, you gain weight. Eating a meal that contains lots of fats and topping it off with a dessert that contains sugar will have the same effect.

There is another nuance to the insulin discussion that must be understood. Certain natural plant foods, such as carrots, are rapidly absorbed, but because they are so low in calories, they do not add weight to your body. A 3½-ounce carrot has about 43 calories and negligible amounts of fat (less than a gram). Who cares if those 43 calories are rapidly absorbed—there are too few of them to matter! On a diet rich in vegetables, including carrots, you consume so few calories that your body will be forced to burn its existing fat supplies to meet its daily energy needs. No one gets fat on carrots.

HOW TO BURN FAT EFFICIENTLY

In general, minimally processed plant foods keep your insulin levels low because they are slowly broken down by your intestines, which means their sugars are released slowly into your bloodstream. So that you can keep burning fat.

Another important point to keep in mind is that the calorie content of your diet is very low when you eat plant foods, even though they are very filling, which forces your body to release stored fat as a fuel source. Even when you eat a plant food that raises insulin levels temporarily because it is rapidly absorbed, such as carrots or fruits, you won't gain weight because these foods are so low in calories. Only carbohydrates that contain concentrated calories that are rapidly absorbed cause weight retention and weight gain.

Controlling your insulin level is critical if you want to lose weight without hunger. The first thing to do is to eat vegetables, beans, fruit, and minimally processed grains, along with low-fat animal foods. Such a diet will keep your daily calorie intake—and your insulin levels—low, which will help your body burn a lot of fat.

But let me show you how processed foods and fat combine to increase your weight, even in meals that are thought to be healthy.

THE TRUTH ABOUT LOW-FAT MEALS

In the 1980s, when the negative effects of fat on health and weight became better known, people started to demand low-fat prepared meals. Unfortunately, when food manufacturers removed the fat from the food, people didn't like the taste, so food processors had to figure out a way to put the fat back into the food, while keeping it low in fat and calories. Some clever industry people put their heads together and came up with a neat little trick that's being used by many manufacturers of prepared food.

One of the more popular prepared dinners is a "heart-healthy" meat loaf. The meal includes meat loaf, succotash, potatoes, and an apple cobbler dessert. Remarkably, this entire meal contains only 320 calories and derives only 25 percent of its calories from fat. How do the food manufacturers manage that? A low-fat, low-calorie meal that looks just like the one Joe's greasy spoon serves.

Well, the secret lies in the dessert. The apple cobbler is composed of apples, sugar, and Grape-Nuts—100 calories, but is entirely fat-free. If we remove the fat-free dessert from the meal, the percentage of calories derived from fat changes dramatically, because fat now makes up more of the meal's total calories. Now we've got a meal of 220 calories, but 80 of them still come from fat. If we divide 80 calories by 220, we find that the meal—minus the dessert—contains 36 percent of its calories from fat, which makes it a high-fat meal. The amount of fat consumed doesn't change. All the food manufacturers did was add fat-free calories so that the fat would be a smaller percentage of the total. In fact, there's nothing "low-fat" or "heart healthy" about this meal. Like shady accountants, the food manufacturers are just juggling the numbers with a little sleight of hand. It's the same meat loaf you get at Joe's greasy spoon (albeit in disguise).

The "heart-healthy" meal has only 320 calories. How did the food manufacturers manage to produce such a low-calorie dinner? Easy. The portions are tiny! It's barely a snack. That little dinner is not going to fill you up for two reasons: first, there's too little there to fill up anyone with an appetite, and second, high-fat foods provide poor satiety. When you're finished, you'll still be hungry. In all likelihood you're going to have two of them. What's more, the concentrated calories from that dessert are rapidly absorbed. They're going to flood your bloodstream with sugars, causing you to store nearly all the fat that's in the meal and to retain the fat in your tissues. People who eat these low-fat, heart-healthy meals don't lose much weight. It's no wonder they're frustrated.

This reminds me of a recent experience while traveling on a large airline. I ordered a low-fat meal and got fettuccine Alfredo made with butter, cream, and eggs—everything you'd expect from a high-fat meal. But the total calories and the total fat were quite low. How'd they do that? I wondered. And then it hit me: minuscule portions! The problem is that when you finish these portion-controlled, low-fat low-calorie meals, you're still hungry, for two reasons: high-fat foods are less filling, and the portions are so tiny that they couldn't fill the stomach of a small child. So you order another one. But when you're done eating, you've consumed lots of calories. If you ate a calorically concentrated dessert, the sugar will be rapidly absorbed, which will ensure that you've stored most of the calories from fat in your tissues. The end result: weight gain.

For Susan, all of this came as a revelation. Not only was she eating foods that were high in protein and fat, but she was eating sugar as well. It's no wonder she was gaining weight, even as she tried to starve herself. The question that still lingered in her mind was, Why do I crave sugar? The answer: The fat instinct.

SUGAR TRIGGERS THE FAT INSTINCT

Sugar is fat's good-looking cousin, but don't let its appeal fool you: it's nearly as bad for weight loss as fat is. Processed carbohydrates, such as sugar, keep you hungry. Two separate studies, one by Barbara J. Rolls, Ph.D., published in the *American Journal of Clinical Nutrition*, and another by P. J. Geiselman, Ph.D., in the journal *Appetite*, each showed that when sugar levels were increased in the diet both appetite and the number of calories consumed increased. After noting that fat "is the macronutrient associated with overeating," Dr. Rolls reported that both sugar and fat "have similar effects on hunger, satiety, and subsequent food intake."

One of the reasons for sugar's propensity for increasing appetite is its ability to raise insulin levels. The higher your insulin levels, the more hungry you are. Also, when people with adult-onset diabetes start taking insulin, their hunger increases dramatically and they usually gain weight.

Processed and refined carbohydrates often lack fiber and water, which means that these foods have little or no bulk. You can eat a lot of them before your stomach's stress receptors tell your brain that it's full and to shut off appetite. Eat a couple of highly refined pastries— the type referred to as "light as a feather"—and you've eaten a few hundred calories before you even notice they're in your stomach. You could eat the box, you tell yourself. Why? Because eating a concentrated-calorie food triggers your fat instinct. The lesson is simple: Once you start eating any form of concentrated calories, your fat instinct makes it very hard to stop.

JOHN WELLES'S STORY

John Welles was one of the pioneers on the Pritikin Program, and, frankly, it was all that stood between him and the grave. John began the program in 1977, after his doctor examined him and told him, flatly, "You don't have many more months to live." He had high blood pressure, gout, insomnia, and was fifty pounds overweight. His cholesterol level was 350 mg/dl and he had coronary heart disease. John had spent the previous four years opening fast-food restaurants—250 of them in all. He rushed to virtually every location to start up each business and be present at grand openings. "I traveled all the time," he said.

He arrived at the Pritikin Center in a wheelchair, exhausted and enfeebled. He was forty-five years old. "That evening I was served chicken pot pie," he said recently. "I remember fishing around, looking for a piece of shredded chicken."

The next morning, he was given his medical examination and told that his exercise program would consist of a single walk around the block each day. That day he did his walk. "A minor miracle," he called it. The next day, he did his once-around-the-block prescription, and then added another round to it. He added an additional trip around the block each day. Meanwhile, he continued to eat the Pritikin diet, and felt stronger with each passing day. At the end of his twenty-eight-day stay at the center, John was walking almost four miles a day.

His health was improving, and his cholesterol levels and weight were falling dramatically. His cholesterol level fell from 350 to 225 mg/dl at the end of his four-week stay at the center. Eventually, it dropped to 180 mg/dl, where it has stayed for the past twenty years. During the months after he began the program, he lost fifty pounds. At 5' 10" tall, John weighs 150 pounds today, and he has never regained the weight in the twenty years he's been on the program.

John begins every morning with a big bowl of oatmeal with bananas, or berries, and nonfat milk. Around 10 A.M., he eats a piece of fruit. At lunch he usually has a large salad, or a plate of vegetables. He takes another fruit break at midafternoon, and has a dinner of steamed vegetables, brown rice, barley, or baked potato. "Every now and then, I eat white rice. I eat a lot of grains." He also enjoys pasta and marinara sauce. Though the Pritikin Program allows animal foods, John has chosen to avoid chicken and turkey. He does enjoy fish, however. Once a week, he cooks a big piece of salmon—"I know that's more than what Pritikin recommends, but what the heck, it's once a week." Along with his salmon, he savors a half bottle of wine ("that's my alcohol quota for the week").

But what is most gratifying to John is that he is healthy and alive. "I really do feel that Nathan Pritikin saved my life. I don't think there's any question that if I hadn't gotten on the program, I wouldn't be here today."

THE FOUR CRITERIA OF A SUCCESSFUL WEIGHT-LOSS PROGRAM

Excessive hunger is the undoing of virtually every other weight-loss program. The reason is that hunger was meant to be uncomfortable, even painful, *so that you would avoid it.* Any program that asks you to limit the size of your meals and go hungry is asking you to defeat Mother Nature. It cannot be done in the long run, and you're going to be mighty frustrated when you try. Hunger triggers the fat instinct, which means that eventually you will gorge on high-fat and calorie-rich foods. Hunger and the fat instinct defeat 95 percent of portion-control dieters. Only those people known as "restrained eaters," who represent a very small percentage of the population, can adhere to portion-control programs. The rest of us simply hate the many discomforts associated with hunger. Moreover, any program that requires you to avoid plant foods, which are the carbohydrate-rich foods, is really asking you to avoid immune-boosting and cancer-fighting nutrition. Following that kind of program will ultimately cost you your health. Either way, you lose.

There are four basic criteria that must be met if a program is to achieve the goals of weight loss, improved health, and sustainability:

1. You must be able to eat until you reach fullness or satiety. In fact, you should be able to avoid chronic hunger entirely, so that you can eat whenever you are hungry, including between meals.

And you must continue to lose weight or maintain your optimal weight.

2. The diet must offer you an abundant supply of nutrition to boost your immune system and promote cancer-fighting functions. It must also be low in fat and cholesterol, since these are the primary causes of disease.

3. You must enjoy the diet. The food has to be filling, delicious, and fully satisfying. It should provide both satiety *and* satisfaction.

4. The program should be adaptable. You should be able to enjoy eating in restaurants, traveling, or socializing with people who do not eat as you do.

Any dietary program that does not meet these four criteria cannot be sustained by most people, and therefore is a waste of time and effort. In this chapter, I've shown you how the Pritikin Program meets the first two criteria for an effective and sustainable program. Our diet allows you to eat until you are full, any time you are hungry. In fact, we encourage you to eat frequently to avoid becoming too hungry and as a way to maintain a low insulin response. The foods that make up our program are low in calories, yet they provide maximum satiety. At the same time, they provide maximum nutrition to support your immune system and cancer-fighting capacities. In chapter 7, I'll show you how you can travel and eat in restaurants and remain on the Pritikin Program, without feeling deprived.

THE BEHAVIORS
THAT OUTSMART
THE FAT INSTINCT

The fat instinct presents us with a classic catch-22: we have to overcome a basic survival mechanism in order to survive. How can we conquer a genetic propensity to eat foods high in fat and sugar, which has been a primary tool of survival throughout human history, so that we can enjoy good health, optimal weight, and, indeed, survive?

The fat instinct continues to dominate us because the foods that keep us in its grip taste good. In order to eat this high-fat diet, however, we must deny its effects on our health and appearance. When you think about it, this is an astounding accomplishment, because scientists have known for decades that the diet that promotes health, abundant energy, optimal weight, and physical beauty is one composed chiefly of fresh vegetables, beans, fruit, whole grains, low-fat animal foods, and nonfat milk. It's the ideal diet from every perspective. It provides maximum nutrition, including the micronutrients that protect you against major diseases, and it fills you up with foods that are low in calories. The problem is that no one wants to eat it!

The fat instinct has created a basic conflict between our desire to enjoy our food and our desire for health and fitness. The challenge we face is to bring the fat instinct and the health instinct back into harmony: to create a diet that promotes health and optimal weight that people actually want to eat—that they actually enjoy eating every day.

Most of the experts who promote a healthful diet have given up trying to create a diet that people actually prefer to eat. Instead, they rely upon people's fear of serious illness, or of premature death, to bring them around to their way of eating. Most people today know that their high-fat, high-cholesterol diets either are contributing to their poor health or are the cause of it. As a result, many of them adopt a diet that relies more heavily on low-fat plant foods. Health proponents keep people on their regimens by using discipline and by promoting the fear that if they return to their old eating patterns their illnesses will return.

At the Pritikin Longevity Center, we know this strategy very well, because we used it for years. My father believed that dietary patterns were culturally instilled, which meant that with sufficient exposure to a new regimen, everyone would learn to enjoy a healthy diet. Only after we had uncovered the fat instinct and its power to influence food choices did we come to a deeper understanding. However, we were then confronted with the challenge of how to outsmart it.

My father used to say that if you want to create a real solution to any problem—one that truly addresses all of the problem's underlying causes—you have to get beyond the limitations of your current thinking, to "break out of the box," and instead ask yourself what characteristics such a solution should possess. Forget about whether or not you can do it.

A program that outsmarts the fat instinct must have two very distinct characteristics. First, it has to create a physiological craving for carbohydrate-rich foods. People have to desire and enjoy the foods that promote optimal weight and health. That's the only way they will be able to stay on the program. Second, the solution must keep the fat instinct dormant. Once people are in the grip of the fat instinct, they have little or no control over their food choices.

So we had to answer two fundamental questions: How do we create a craving for carbohydrate-rich foods so that people actually enjoy foods that create fullness on the fewest number of calories? And, how do we keep the fat instinct at bay, especially in the modern world, in which it is being endlessly stimulated?

We created a program that accomplishes both of these goals. Our program creates a craving in people for the foods that promote health, and consequently results in optimal weight, abundant energy, and enhanced appearance, without relying on people's willingness to go hungry or constantly feel deprived. It also keeps the fat instinct dormant, so that you can enjoy eating a diet that promotes health, without having to be constantly burdened by cravings for fat and calorie-rich foods.

One of the surprising and welcome discoveries we made as we implemented this program at the Pritikin Longevity Center is that it allows people to make less-than-optimal choices on occasion and still maintain their health. The program itself creates a certain amount of flexibility.

SHAPING TRADITIONAL BEHAVIOR TO FIT A MODERN LIFESTYLE

We realized that you cannot take the traditional human diet, apply it to the modern lifestyle, and expect people to adhere to it. It doesn't work. With its emphasis on rich foods and sedentary behaviors, the modern lifestyle promotes the fat instinct, and thereby triggers an endless craving for foods that contribute to overweight and illness. The fat instinct also *biologically limits your capacity to eat carbohydrates*. This revelation changed our entire program. We realized that behaviors that we had previously thought were unrelated to diet actually influence the kinds of foods you desire.

Certain behaviors make each of us crave the foods the human body was designed to eat, and in the process they outsmart the fat instinct. Remarkably, these behaviors combine to create an overall effect on your body, especially your palate. The more you practice these behaviors, the more powerful their impact is on your dietary choices and health. Not surprisingly, the behaviors that outsmart the fat instinct were—and still are—fundamental to a traditional way of life.

In chapter 1, I described the way of life our early ancestors followed. That pattern amounted to daily scavenging, gathering, and hunting for food, and reliance upon plant foods as the primary source of calories, with occasional supplementation from animal foods. This pattern is ingrained in the human species; indeed, it even served to shape our biological and genetic makeup. Within this pattern are the keys to overcoming the fat instinct and establishing good health, optimal weight, and abundant energy.

Our ancestors didn't have to worry about calories or weight loss or whether or not they ate enough plant foods on any given day. They just lived instinctually and ate the foods nature provided. Today, living in the modern world, we have infinitely more choices available to us, which means that we can no longer live by instinct alone. Patterns of behavior that long ago were unconscious and imposed upon us by the environment must now be practiced consciously if we are to achieve optimal health.

Of course, I'm not suggesting that you should scavenge instead of shop, or dig up potatoes from your garden and eat them while sitting on the ground. What I am suggesting is that we take the old traditional pattern and modernize it. Specifically, there are five behaviors that were fundamental to our ancestors' way of life that we can adopt today. These five behaviors create a cascade of physiological and psychological changes within you, so that once you adopt the first behavior, and then follow it with the second, third, fourth, and fifth, the biochemical changes occur with a certain momentum. Soon you will find yourself craving carbohydrate foods, losing weight, and restoring your health, vitality, and physical appearance without any sense of hunger or deprivation. The more you practice these behaviors, the more momentum you build, so that as the craving for healthy foods becomes stronger, the benefits that impact your daily life become more pronounced and occur more rapidly. In a very short time, your body begins to tell you that you're doing the right things, because the changes are releasing you from the malaise and debilitation caused by the fat instinct. Your health instinct, which is continually creating a yearning for good health, abundant energy, and enhanced physical appearance, is being strengthened and rewarded.

These five behaviors are synergistic, meaning that the effect of all five combined is greater than the effect of each behavior practiced alone. I will show you how each behavior actually produces the need for the next.

1. EXERCISE

Our food cravings and food preferences are determined in part by how much physical activity we engage in each day. You can be made to crave carbohydrate-rich foods, and in the process transform your tastes, simply by doing a relatively small amount of exercise each day, such as taking a daily walk.

Most of us think that our food cravings emerge from some mysterious quarter of the psyche over which we have no control. We tend to think of exercise as an uncomfortable and sometimes even painful activity that's good for our muscular, skeletal, and cardiovascular systems. We don't connect these two fundamental aspects of life: diet and activity. However, if you live a sedentary life, you will tend to prefer fat and calorie-rich foods and resist carbohydrate-rich foods.

On the other hand, if you walk as little as two miles a day over what you normally do in the course of your daily activity you will crave more carbohydrate-rich foods, and in the process find yourself preferring the very foods that promote health, optimal weight, and abundant energy.

How and Where the Body Stores Energy

We store about 1,500 calories of energy from carbohydrates in our muscles and liver. Compare that to the 100,000 calories of energy most lean people store as fat, and the 200,000 to 300,000 calories overweight people keep tucked away in their tissues. Obviously, there's a lot more fat than carbohydrate stored in your tissues. If you burn a fuel mix that's 50 percent carbohydrate and 50 percent fat, you're going to burn up your carbohydrate stores long before you put a dent in your fat reserves. Since your body relies almost exclusively on carbohydrates as a fuel for brain function and rapid physical action, it is going to demand that you replace carbohydrate stores the next time you eat. In fact, the more you exercise, the more your body demands that you eat carbohydrates. A food craving is the way the body makes such a demand. All of a sudden, carbohydrate-rich foods are going to look good to you and taste good, too.

Think of your muscles as your carbohydrate-fuel tank. That tank is tiny in comparison to your fat tank, which means even small amounts of exercise will deplete the tank and force you to fill up again and again on carbohydrate-rich foods to give your body the fuel it needs. Thus, by regularly depleting your carbohydrate storage tanks, you maintain an ongoing craving for carbohydrate-rich foods. Once this occurs, and you start to correctly follow your cravings, you naturally lose weight.

The Paradox of Exercise and Weight Loss

You might be surprised to learn that those who exercise not only lose weight initially, but also stand the greatest chance of keeping that weight off, especially if they combine their weight-loss program with appropriate diet. On the other hand, the vast majority of people who use diet alone to lose weight fail to keep the weight off for even a year after they started their programs.

But here's an interesting fact: *Exercise alone is not a very efficient way to lose weight.* You burn about 100 calories per mile of walking or jogging. There are 3,500 calories in every pound of fat. That means that you have to walk thirty-five miles just to burn 3,500 calories; but remember, only half of the calories you burn are from fat. The other half are from carbohydrates. That means that you've got to walk seventy miles to lose a full pound of fat. That's pretty discouraging, if you ask me. Yet, those who exercise lose weight and have the best chance of keeping it off. Why? Because exercise naturally changes people's food preferences—they start to crave carbohydrate-rich foods, such as fruits, vegetables, and grains—and those new food choices result in weight loss. Such changes often occur unconsciously; people are not even aware that they are changing their diets. They're just following instinctual cravings. Yet, the new food choices, brought about by the exercise, change everything.

How Exercise Influences Food Cravings

A recent study done on rats tested the effects exercise had on the foods that dieting animals craved.

A population of rats was given inadequate amounts of food every ay. They quickly became irritable and hungry. Half the rats were made to exercise. The other half were allowed to lie around and relax, just as many of us do when we're hungry and irritable. After several weeks, the two groups of rats were allowed to eat from two food troughs, one that contained high-fat foods and the other that contained high-carbohydrate foods. The rats could eat as much as they wanted from each trough. Researchers studied the rats' dietary choices and recorded the percentage of calories they ate from fat versus carbohydrate.

The results were interesting: The sedentary rats ate 50 percent of their calories from fat, while the exercising rats ate only 32 percent of their calories from fat. The researchers repeated the study. This time, the couch-potato rats ate a diet that was composed of 70 percent fat, while the exercising rats continued to eat a diet of only 32 percent fat. In other words, the diet of the sedentary rats actually got worse, while that of the exercising rats remained relatively low in fat and high in carbohydrates. Clearly, the researchers were able to influence the kinds of nutrients the rats craved by altering a single factor: exercise.

Researchers believe the two groups craved different foods because exercise caused one group of rats to deplete their carbohydrate stores, forcing them to replenish carbohydrates the minute they were allowed to eat. The sedentary rats did not deplete their carbohydrate reserves significantly and therefore had less need for carbohydrates once they were allowed to eat.

A lot of people argue that food cravings are so influenced by culture that it's hard to know what the basis of any craving may be. This is why this rat study is so interesting: unlike humans, rats are immune to cultural influences, such as television commercials and motivational talks, that might affect the kinds of foods they want to eat. Rats are going to eat what's available, or, if they have a choice, they're going to eat what they prefer—no matter what's on TV.

The changes that occurred in the rats are consistent with those discovered in human research as well. At Stanford University, Peter Wood, Ph.D., examined a group of middle-aged men who jogged daily for two years. The group was given no nutritional advice or encouragement to change their diets. Wood carefully monitored their food choices. One of the interesting findings was that their appetite increased significantly from the exercise, which is not unexpected when you consider that lumberjacks eat about 5,000 calories a day and triathletes about 8,000 calories a day. Nevertheless, the extra calories consumed by the joggers were primarily from carbohydrates. Moreover, the joggers lost weight. Wood concluded that exercise creates a craving for carbohydrates, while sedentary lifestyles promote the desire for fat.

A large study involving nearly thirty thousand people that was done by E. J. Simoes and his colleagues replicated Wood's findings. Simoes found that the more people exercised, the more they ate carbohydrates, no matter whether they were men or women. The more sedentary the participants' lifestyles, the more they ate fatty foods.

A survey of 1,837 women runners published in *The New England Journal of Medicine* (1996; 334:1298–303) found a direct correlation between the number of miles the women ran and the amount of fruit they ate. The longer the distance they ran per week, the more fruit they ate each week.

People whose physical exercise levels range from moderate to highly active were found to eat more fiber, less total fat, and less saturated fat than sedentary participants, according to a study done by S. Boyd Eaton, M.D. The active people also consumed more foods rich in vitamins (A, C, D, E), beta carotene, and calcium, and ate more fruits and vegetables.

Exercise Regulates Our Desire for Carbohydrates

Some scientists who observed that people who exercise actually eat better made the argument that exercisers are part of a select population who tend to take better care of their health across the board. Only recently did researchers gain the understanding that food preferences are changed by exercise. Exercise increases the body's need for carbohydrates. Because the body has a limited capacity to store them, we have to keep filling up on carbohydrates to meet the body's demands. As everyone knows, a small gas tank requires lots of refills. If, by exercising, you keep lowering your carbohydrate reserves, you're going to need lots of refills, which means you're going to crave carbohydrates. But if you don't exercise, your body will limit the amount of carbohydrate foods you can safely eat.

In a groundbreaking review of the literature reported in the *American Journal of Clinical Nutrition* (1995; 62:820–36), J. P. Flatt, Ph.D., revealed that the body has mechanisms for regulating carbohydrate consumption based on how much energy you are burning each day. If you suddenly try to increase carbohydrate consumption without burning more energy through exercise, your body will first increase metabolism to burn off the excess carbohydrates, and then decrease your appetite for carbohydrates.

Let's say you want to adopt a diet rich in plant foods and you do not exercise. You're suddenly going to increase the amount of carbohydrates in your bloodstream. Your body is going to say, "Wait a minute, I don't need all those carbs, because I've got plenty stored up in my muscles and liver." It will therefore resist taking extra carbohydrates. The body says to itself, "I don't want any more carbohydrates! I want protein or fat." In a very real sense, a lifestyle without exercise maintains the fat instinct's grip on your consciousness and your behavior, which means you will constantly be directed to high-fat foods just like the sedentary rats were. Moreover, as long as the fat instinct is guiding your actions and your biochemistry, your body resists consuming carbohydrate-rich foods in any significant quantities, which means you will have great difficulty changing your diet and behavior.

On a Sedentary Lifestyle, a Healthy Diet Is a Pipe Dream for Most

During the past twenty years, lots of people have tried to increase their carbohydrates without increasing their exercise. Unfortunately, this strategy can have adverse effects on health.

If you discipline yourself to eat a high-carbohydrate diet, but don't exercise enough, the excess carbohydrates you eat can be converted to triglycerides, or fats, in your liver, and then flood your bloodstream with tiny globules of fat. Elevated triglycerides can lower high-density lipoproteins, or HDLs, the "good" cholesterol that reduces your risk of heart disease.

The leading health agencies, including the National Academy of Sciences, the National Cancer Institute, and the U.S. Department of

Health and Human Services, recommend that Americans eat at least five servings of fresh fruits and vegetables per day, and at least six servings of grains and beans per day. Most Americans are lucky if they get three servings of vegetables or fruit per day, and one serving of grains (as bread), and even these are usually processed. One reason we can't comply with the recommendations, of course, is because most Americans are sedentary.

The less energy we expend, the more carbohydrates remain stored in our muscles and liver. Consequently, we have no real appetite for carbohydrate-rich foods. It's difficult to return to the human diet without increasing our daily energy expenditure, which means we must exercise.

Based on the available data and our knowledge of how many carbohydrate-calories are expended during exercise, we can figure out how many more servings of plant foods a person will desire if he or she increases exercise to, say, two miles of walking per day. If you have been sedentary, but start walking two miles per day, you will find it easier to add two servings of vegetables and one serving of fresh fruit per day. The study shows that the more you exercise, the more fruits and vegetables you will eat, making it more likely that you will consume the recommended amounts of plant foods each day. You would be well on your way to enjoying all the health benefits of the Pritikin Program.

It's very important to understand what I mean by exercise. At the outset, I'm really talking only about walking or some other physical activity that will expend your carbohydrate reserves, at least four times per week. So, if you are currently living a sedentary life but begin walking just two miles a day—which for most people requires only a half hour—your body will demand that you increase carbohydrates significantly. Ideally, you should exercise from four to six times each week. Taking a two-mile walk is plenty if you are currently sedentary, and you do not have to walk fast. A stroll is fine. The distance you walk is more important than how fast you walk it. You should increase your exercise over time. The more you exercise, the stronger your craving for carbohydrates will become.

At the Pritikin Longevity Center, we have observed firsthand the power of exercise to change people's palates and their food preferences. For years, we have welcomed new people to our center on Sunday. In the past, every new participant would receive a complete physical and treadmill stress test on Monday and Tuesday, which would indicate how much exercise he or she could participate in. Only on Wednesday did everyone start exercising at his or her own level. We noted for years that people enjoyed the food on our program so much more after Wednesday. Initially, we thought that it had to do with the menus presented after Wednesday, so we changed the menus to provide the foods people enjoyed the most on Monday and Tuesday. No change. People uniformly enjoyed our foods better after Wednesday, which had us scratching our heads for years. And then the research came out demonstrating that exercise creates a preference for carbohydrate-rich foods. After that, we had all our doctors come into the center to conduct physicals on the weekends and had everyone exercising on Monday morning. The results have been phenomenal. We have more people reporting that they immediately enjoy the food than ever before. We've also got more people coming back to our center for tune-ups, refreshers, or cooking classes than we ever had, just as we have more local alumni from the Los Angeles area coming back for meals at night.

Exercise can change your food preferences and diet. But once you start exercising and begin craving carbohydrate-rich foods, you must choose your foods wisely in order to lose weight and improve your health. Thus, the first step creates a demand for the second.

2. CHOOSE THE RIGHT CARBOHYDRATE

Once you begin exercising and start craving more carbohydrates, you'll have won a great victory. You have set yourself up to enjoy the Pritikin Program, restore your health, enjoy great vitality, and optimal weight. But once you start exercising regularly and craving carbohydrates, there is the danger of eating the wrong kinds.

As we have already seen, carbohydrates come in many forms. You can satisfy your carbohydrate craving with ice cream (which contains lots of sugars and fat) or with bakery products, such as pastries, doughnuts, or muffins, all of which contain both processed carbohydrates and fat. The combination of processed carbohydrates and fat can cause you to gain weight, even if you are exercising.

Remember the Lissner study I reported in chapter 3, in which the fat was hidden in common foods such as muffins? The subjects in that study never knew how much fat they were eating, even though a lot of their foods—especially the flour products—were high-fat bombs. Baked flour products often contain fat, but the fat is hidden so effectively that you would never know it was there by taste alone. Hidden fat triggers your fat instinct and causes you to overeat and gain weight.

This is precisely where most people go wrong when they start exercising: they start craving carbohydrates, but they don't discern the difference between plant foods and processed carbohydrates. In our modern culture, a craving for carbohydrates can lead you directly to fat.

A Simple Rule of Thumb to Guide You

Here's a simple guideline for choosing the right carbohydrate-rich food: Eat the plant-based food that provides the maximum fullness, or satiety, with the fewest possible calories. Choose a plant food—a vegetable, fruit, bean, or whole grain—that is closest to its natural state. With very few exceptions, plant foods that have undergone little or no processing will fill you up and provide you with very few calories. Low in fat and calories, but loaded with nutrition and bulk, they will encourage weight loss without triggering feelings of deprivation.

Some examples of foods that provide the maximum fullness with the fewest possible calories are potatoes and sweet potatoes; oatmeal; fruit; a wide assortment of green, leafy, orange, and yellow vegetables; lentils and other beans; vegetable-based soups; and brown rice and other whole grains. (In chapter 7, I provide a three-step program for choosing maximum-satiety, low-calorie foods, along with menus, fast-food ideas, and snacks.)

Steer clear of processed foods, especially those containing fat. These foods will be less filling and will have an abundance of calories. That means, of course, that you will eat more of them before you're satisfied and, consequently, add fat to your body. Obvious examples

of processed plant foods that have added fat are cakes, cookies, croissants, doughnuts, and muffins.

Nature produces foods that are either high in fat or high in carbohydrates, no matter whether the food source is a plant or an animal.
The only exception is milk, which contains both carbohydrates and fat
to support the rapid growth of infants. Only processed foods, which
are made by humans, have *both* fat and carbohydrates in significant
quantities. Some processed foods are low in calories and fat, and fill
you up. Both pasta and oatmeal are healthful choices if you want to
lose weight without feeling hungry.

The Pritikin eating plan is not a vegetarian regimen. It includes
plenty of low-fat animal foods, but plant-based carbohydrate foods are
the keys to weight loss and good health. Our program relies on them
to provide low-calorie, filling foods with abundant nutrition.

Good Food Choices + Exercise = Flexibility

Any program that does not allow an occasional digression isn't a
program people can stick with for life (and isn't one that I could
follow myself). Fortunately, people who adopt the Pritikin Program
have some built-in protective mechanisms that allow them to eat a
processed food from time to time without having to worry about
gaining weight. The reason for this is regular exercise, which allows
your muscles to store the carbohydrates flooding your bloodstream.
The result is that your body goes right on burning fat.

People who lead sedentary lives can't store excess carbohydrates,
because their muscles are loaded with glycogen. The minute they eat
a processed food, even one that does not contain fat, their storage
tanks are overwhelmed with a flood of excess carbohydrates. Their
bodies are forced to burn the excess immediately, which means that
fat burning is shut off. All the fat in their tissues is retained, along
with any fat that may be in their food.

The best advice is to eat unprocessed plant foods, but you do not
have to be perfect to enjoy the benefits the Pritikin Program provides.

In the next chapter, you'll find that our diet is divided into three different steps, each one based on high-satiety, low-fat foods. Each step

allows slightly different amounts of fat and processed carbohydrates. As you become adept at preparing these foods and ordering them in restaurants, you will realize that you can eat healthfully under virtually any condition. I've even included guidelines for those times when you want to relax and enjoy a meal that is outside the optimal guidelines. If you become knowledgeable about the Pritikin Program, and all the choices you have available to you in restaurants and at social occasions, you will find that you have the flexibility to remain on the Pritikin Program forever, without any self-imposed hunger. Indeed, you will experience firsthand that these are the foods you actually desire.

3. LIMIT YOUR FAT INTAKE

By taking the first two steps of the program, you have created a craving for carbohydrates and are selecting the right carbohydrate foods. These steps alone will help to promote optimal weight and good health. You have met the first criterion for a true solution to the fat instinct: You have created a desire for the foods that will give you the results you want.

But you still have to meet the second criterion, which is to keep the fat instinct dormant. You've got to dampen the influence of the fat instinct so that it does not control your cravings and food choices. The first step in reducing the influence of the fat instinct is to limit fat intake. Fat consumption alone causes the arousal of the fat instinct, which in turn demands that you eat fat and calorie-rich foods.

As I have pointed out, eating foods rich in fat contributes to the onset of major diseases, as well as to overweight and obesity. The primary sources of fat in the modern world are animal foods, such as red meat, eggs, and whole milk products; processed foods that contain fat; seeds and nuts; and oils, such as corn, olive, safflower, and sesame.

Humans have always had to limit their fat consumption. But our early ancestors had an advantage over us: nature limited the amount of fat available to them. Because the availability of animal food was sporadic at best, plant foods had to be relied on for daily calories and nutrition. The animal foods available were low in fat. Consequently, our ancestors could eat as much fat as they could lay their hands on and still maintain a low-fat diet.

In the modern world we do not have those same natural protections. Indeed, our society encourages us to overeat fat whenever and wherever we have the opportunity. And, unfortunately, the supply of fat is unlimited. We have fallen into a destructive relationship with the fat instinct in which there are no natural checks and balances.

If we are to sustain our health and survive the current conditions, our environment demands that we create certain limits on fat consumption ourselves. The first two steps in this program assist you in doing just that. First, exercise causes you to crave carbohydrate-rich foods; second, choosing the right carbohydrate allows you to fill up on low-calorie foods. A sense of fullness, or satiety, alone diminishes the influence of the fat instinct, because you have signaled your brain that you have adequate calories to survive. Just as hunger is one of the biggest triggers of the fat instinct, fullness is one of the most powerful tools for outsmarting it.

Eat as Little Fat as Possible

How much fat should you have? The Pritikin Program has historically recommended eating up to $3^1/_2$ ounces of animal foods per day, along with two small servings of skim milk or nonfat cheese. But you can answer the question of how much fat *you* should eat by asking yourself how much weight you want to lose and what you want your blood cholesterol level to be.

Your blood cholesterol level is largely determined by the amount of saturated fat in your diet. Saturated fat is found mostly in animal foods. Your weight is affected by all forms of fat, including saturated, monounsaturated (found in olives and olive oil), and polyunsaturated (derived from vegetable oils). If your cholesterol is high, you should probably avoid all saturated fats. If you are overweight, you should limit or avoid all forms of added fat.

In the next chapter, I'll give you the details of the Pritikin eating plan, as well as our Stepping Program that will allow you to eat more fat initially as you progress toward your optimal amount of fat consumption. This program can also be used to guide you in situations that require you to make less-than-optimal choices, such as in restaurants or while traveling.

In any case, we encourage you to eat minimal amounts of animal foods in combination with larger amounts of high-satiety plant foods, which will give you a sense of fullness and satisfaction long before you trigger your fat instinct and consume too many calories. But our program goes a giant step further. We encourage you to eat frequently, as many as six times per day. The effects of frequent eating on weight loss and health are profound.

4. Eat Frequently to Avoid Hunger and Burn Fat

Eating several times during the course of the day accomplishes two fundamental goals, both of which support weight loss and optimal health: First, you aren't hungry all the time, which means that the fat instinct slumbers. Second, you keep your insulin levels low, *which keeps you burning more fat all day long, even as you eat throughout the day.*

Our ancestors ate as many as twelve or more servings of vegetables and fruits per day. On a good day, they were eating all day long. The average American eats only two meals a day. This way of eating promotes weight retention and weight gain.

Most Americans skip breakfast entirely, or simply have a cup or two of coffee. Some eat a processed roll with their coffee. Hamburgers and sandwiches that include luncheon meats or tuna and mayonnaise are the most popular lunch items; of course, they contain both fat and processed carbohydrates (the bread). One of the most common side dishes is French fries, a processed carbohydrate food that's loaded with fat-calories. Along with this lunch, most of us have a sugary soft drink. At dinner, we typically eat a big meal that usually includes both a form of meat and processed carbohydrates. Hence, a typical day's food consists mostly of protein, fat, and processed foods. The effect of this combination is to rapidly raise insulin levels, retain the fat that is on our body, and store the fat that is in the meal. Weight gain is virtually inevitable.

In chapter 1, we saw Frank do what so many Americans do today: skip meals in the belief that he would lose weight, when in fact all he did was increase hunger, trigger his fat instinct, and bring on a binge. Skipping meals encourages gorging. When Frank skipped breakfast and ate a small lunch, he was ravenous by dinnertime. If he succeeded in eating only a small portion at dinner, he was miserable all night long. He soon found out that such a pattern cannot be sustained. What did he end up doing? He gorged, causing fat and processed carbohydrates to flood his bloodstream and add weight to his body. He learned that eating infrequently often results in weight gain—even while you are starving yourself—because it triggers the fat instinct.

On the other hand, eating more frequently, as our ancestors did, outsmarts the fat instinct, because we are never forced to feel hungry, which means that our survival instincts are not aroused.

Eating low-satiety foods—those that include fat and processed carbohydrates—will cause you to eat high-calorie meals, thereby limiting the number of meals you eat each day. On the other hand, if you eat high-satiety meals composed of low-calorie, high-fiber foods, you will feel compelled to eat frequently—*even while you lose weight.*

Eat Frequently to Lose Weight

The combination of high-fat, processed carbohydrates and high insulin will promote weight gain. But recently researcher David Jenkins, Ph.D., asked a very simple question: What happens to insulin levels when you portion out the same quantity of food over numerous meals? Jenkins compared the effects of two types of eating patterns on insulin. He began by having volunteers, all of whom were diabetic, eat three meals a day of a diet consisting of 30 percent fat. He then monitored their insulin levels. Predictably, their blood sugar and insulin levels went up and remained high, which reduces fat burning and increases fat storage. Then Jenkins took the same people, placed them on the same diet, but portioned out the food in thirteen small meals, taken every hour. The result was that insulin levels remained low throughout the day. In fact, the people who ate thirteen small meals throughout the day produced 30 percent less insulin per day than those who ate the three large meals each day, even though they were both on the exact same diet.

One reason the insulin stayed low was that less sugar hit the blood from the smaller meals than from the big meals. The lower blood sugar levels naturally kept insulin levels down. But there was another reason for the low insulin levels: the sugar hitting the blood at any given time was not enough to overwhelm the storage capacity of the liver and muscles, which meant that less insulin was needed to keep blood sugar levels low. Jenkins and others demonstrated that when you eat frequent meals throughout the day, insulin levels are kept low and fat burning continues.

On the Pritikin Program, you are encouraged to eat six times a day. It's easier than you think, because at least three of those meals are essentially healthy snacks that can be eaten at your desk at work or at home in the evening. The effect of increasing your meal frequency—especially when eating low-calorie plant foods—is significant weight loss, without ever going hungry. Also, by eating frequent meals, we keep the fat instinct at bay. We eat when we're hungry, and thus do not trigger our biological need to gorge on fat.

At the Pritikin Longevity Center, people eat breakfast between 7 and 8 A.M.; a snack around 10 A.M.; lunch at noon; a snack around 2 or 2:30 P.M.; dinner between 6 and 7 P.M.; and a snack at night. This is one of the ways we conquer the fat instinct at the center: we give people plenty of food that is delicious, low in fat, and filling. We do not want people to be excessively hungry, because hunger will incite their fat instinct and defeat the program. Despite the fact that people are satisfied and full, they lose weight, their cholesterol levels fall, and they feel good.

Our program tries to recreate the nutritional environment and the eating patterns of our ancestors. Eating frequently throughout the day prevents hunger and encourages weight loss.

5. BE CONSISTENT

Our ancestors ate the foods that nature provided them with. In fact, nature offered a highly varied menu that changed according to the season. In the spring and summer months, nature gave an abundance of plant foods: edible leaves and soft shoots, potatoes and other ubers, and plump fruits. In the fall and winter, roots, berries, seeds, and nuts were widely available. Seeds and nuts provided our ancestors with additional fat to fortify their calories reserves against the hardships of winter. The fall and winter also provided an abundance of animal foods, as animals gathered in large herds and migrated to warmer and more hospitable climes. These animals also tended to be fatter themselves, as they added calories to their bodies in order to endure the famines of winter.

Each season provided its own distinct food supply. Consequently, our ancestors had to adapt their gathering and hunting strategies to the particular food being offered by nature. They had to adapt their palates not only to enjoy the kinds of foods that were available but also to survive. They had to want to eat the food. For example, seeds and nuts appear in the autumn and winter. If Paleolithic man was driven by a wild and implacable craving for nuts in March, he might pass up the potatoes, leeks, and edible roots that nature was offering, and consequently starve to death. Adaptation of the palate was a survival mechanism. As long as people yearned for what was available, they didn't waste calories of energy searching for food that wasn't.

Today, we don't have that problem. Food choices are no longer regulated by the seasons; therefore, having to adapt our palates to a particular kind of food is considered a hardship. One of the advantages our ancestors had over us is that they were forced to eat a particular set of foods consistently throughout a particular season, which gave their palates sufficient exposure to a certain set of flavors so that adaptation could take place. Soon they found themselves enjoying the foods they were eating.

This same phenomenon can take place within each of us, as well, if we are given the right circumstances to change. As with our ancestors, when we maintain a particular diet consistently over time, we come to enjoy the new set of flavors, just as much as we did those of our previous diet.

This adaptation was demonstrated at the Monell Chemical Senses Institute in Philadelphia, where Dr. Richard Mattes discovered that when people were asked to refrain from eating fat, and fat-substitute foods, they naturally came to enjoy foods that were low in fat. He compared two groups of people, both of which had previously eaten a high-fat diet, but were now instructed to eat a diet that contained between 15 and 20 percent of its calories from fat. One group did not eat any fat-substitute foods, and consequently avoided the sensory experience of fat entirely. The other group was allowed to eat fat-substitute foods. Mattes found that after twelve weeks, the group that had avoided fat and fat-substitute foods adapted to, and came to enjoy, their low-fat diet. In fact, they no longer missed the sensory experience or the flavor of fat. They reported enjoying their diets as much as those who were allowed to eat the fat-substitute foods.

Mattes cited skim milk as one of many examples of low-fat foods that people had come to prefer over their high-fat counterparts. At the outset of the study, the participants routinely drank whole milk, which contains 50 percent of its calories from fat. But after twelve weeks on the low-fat diet, the participants preferred the low-fat skim milk over whole milk. In fact, many people have changed their taste buds to prefer skim milk over whole milk, even though they initially found skim milk to be a slightly repulsive form of "blue water."

Mattes's study demonstrates that when we avoid high-fat foods, as well as the sensory experience of fat, we come to enjoy a new set of flavors and sensory pleasures. In effect, we repeat the experience of our ancestors. The key to such adaptation is consistency.

The power of consistency to change our preference for flavors was demonstrated by a long-term study called MRFIT (Multiple Risk Factor Intervention Trial), in which twelve thousand people were followed from 1973 to 1982 to see what effects, if any, changes in diet and smoking would have on their rates of heart disease. Six thousand of those people were educated to change their eating habits to lower fat and cholesterol, and to stop smoking, while the other six thousand, called the control group, were given no such education. A recent analysis of the data emerging from MRFIT (reported in the *Journal of Clinical Nutrition*) has demonstrated the power of consistency to improve health. People who reported that they "seldom" deviate from the dietary recommendations given to them by nutritionists as part of the study had the greatest reductions in blood cholesterol levels. Those who said they "frequently" deviated from the recommendations had only half the drop in blood cholesterol than those who "seldom" deviated. Those who said they "always" deviate had the smallest drop in cholesterol. Blood cholesterol levels are directly related to how much fat and cholesterol we consume as part of our daily diets. As blood cholesterol goes up, so too do the rates of heart attack, stroke, high blood pressure, and cancer. Thus, the more consistent people were on their diet, the greater their results. Those who strayed could not adhere to the more healthful diet.

SYNERGY IS THE KEY TO SUCCESS

Each of the five steps has a distinct influence on our food preferences and the fat instinct, but none of them alone has the power to transform your palate and your health that all of them have when used together. The whole is greater than the sum of its parts, and that is certainly the case with the Pritikin Program. If you exercise at least four or five times per week, choose the right carbohydrates, limit your fat intake, and eat frequently, your fat instinct will remain dormant, which means you will not crave fatty foods. At that point, you will be able to consciously limit your intake of fat and calorie-rich foods. And if you maintain consistency, you will experience dramatic results, while you thoroughly enjoy the Pritikin Eating Plan.

Combining all five behaviors has the same effect as a snowball rolling down a mountain: it gets bigger as it gains momentum, just as the effects of these five behaviors become more pronounced as we follow them together.

The U.S. Department of Agriculture provided researchers with nutritional, exercise, and medical information obtained from 5,484 volunteers. The scientists found that people who reported being concerned about both their diet and exercise patterns were 49 percent less likely to be overweight than people who were sedentary. Interestingly, people who reported being concerned about only one of these two health promoters were only 19 percent less likely to be overweight than those who were sedentary.

The fact is that people who exercise tend to eat better, as long as they know which type of carbohydrate to choose—plant foods in their natural state, as opposed to processed carbohydrates. As long as you choose plant foods, you cannot help but achieve your optimal weight, look years younger than you are, lower your risk factors for disease, and enjoy abundant energy.

In 1997, scientists reported the largest survey of people who had successfully lost weight and kept that weight off for five years. Researchers conducted the study by gathering a group of 784 people who had lost an average of 66 pounds and then simply asked them how they lost the weight and how they kept it off for at least five years. More than 90 percent of these people responded that they had increased their exercise habits. But exercise alone was not sufficient to lose the weight, they said. Eighty-nine percent said that they also changed their diets, specifically reducing fat consumption.

Actually, the amount of exercise they did in addition to their normal daily activities—those related to work, for example—was not all that much. On average, these people walked approximately 14 miles per week, or about two miles per day. However, that small amount of exercise was accompanied by substantial changes in diet. Both the men and the women brought their fat intake down below 30 percent of their total calories—the men to 23 percent of total calories and the women to 25 percent. Remarkably, 33 percent of the group brought their fat intake down below 20 percent of their total calories. We can safely surmise that they replaced their high-fat animal foods with low-fat plant foods, such as grains, vegetables, and fruits.

Yet, they did not starve themselves while they lost the weight and kept it off. On average, the study participants reported eating five meals per day!

Was their remarkable ability to keep their weight off difficult? the researchers asked. No, the vast majority said. Sixty-eight percent told the researchers that weight maintenance was "easy" or "moderately easy." Only 32 percent said it was "hard."

Yet, the impact of these changes on their lives was substantial. No less than 85 percent of them said that the changes in diet and exercise and the resulting weight loss boosted their self-confidence, energy levels, general mood, physical health, and overall quality of life.

It's important to stress that the Pritikin Program is not a rigid set of rules, but an approach to good health based on the five behaviors I have described. By implementing these five principles every day, you will naturally improve your health, lower your weight, and provide long-lasting and optimal energy.

A PROGRAM THAT ALLOWS YOU TO HAVE FOIBLES

One of the things that I enjoy the most about following the Pritikin Program is that it allows me to be human. I don't have to be perfect in order to enjoy the benefits of the Pritikin way of life. Frankly, I have no interest in being rigid or perfect. I'd rather enjoy life. If you apply the five behaviors I have outlined every day, you will be able to indulge your sweet tooth from time to time, or eat a little more of those fat-free cookies that you particularly like. People who apply the principles of the Pritikin Program enjoy not only good health, but also greater latitude in all kinds of situations they face each day.

Health is the goal we are shooting for, but we also want to enjoy ourselves each day as we reach for that goal. Our program creates the conditions for you to enjoy the foods that fill you up and promote health. And it delivers on its promises. It mimics the way of life that is consistent with our genes, a way of life that harmonizes and balances the fat and health instincts. Ancient humans ate approximately twelve servings of vegetables and fruits per day, according to research conducted by S. Boyd Eaton, M.D., one of the world's leading authorities on Paleolithic nutrition. Consider for a moment how much energy it required to discover a single wild potato. That alone could take a good deal of walking or running, searching the ground, probing, and digging, all the while keeping alert for any wild beasts that might attack. Once they ate their food, they had to look for more. Searching for food alone was a workout. Our ancestors "exercised," ate the right kind of carbohydrates, ate frequently, and maintained their diets consistently. Consequently, their palates adapted and they came to enjoy the foods they ate, which supported their survival.

The Pritikin Program attempts to modernize the human pattern, or human lifestyle. Each of us must recover something from the ancient human past if we are to enjoy health, vitality, optimal weight, and enhanced physical appearance in the present. Indeed, when we consider the effects of the fat instinct on our health and longevity, we come to realize that the traditional lifestyle is essential for our survival as well.

SUSAN'S VICTORY

Perhaps because Susan was a veteran of so many dietary approaches, she was just a bit skeptical of our program, at least at first. Still, it wasn't long after she had heard all the lectures and started exercising and enjoying the food that she saw the weight come off her body as it had never come off before. One of the differences, Susan realized, was simple: "I didn't have to go hungry or feel run down to follow the program. When I made a mistake or went off the program for a day, it didn't collapse all at once, which is what happened on my high-protein or portion-control diets. In fact, I realized that hunger was a big part of why I had failed at every other diet. I hated being hungry and having no energy. Something about being hungry made me irritable and even angry. It seemed like my body had turned against me. It wouldn't work properly. I had to starve myself to keep my weight down, and that made me obsessed with food. But as soon as I started the Pritikin Program, I realized that it is really important for me to eat whenever I am hungry. I have to do that to feel good. What was amazing to me was that as I ate, I was losing weight. I walk every day. I have my stepping program, which gives me choices in all kinds of situations. And the best part of it all is that I've lost thirty-five pounds and I feel better than I've felt since I was in college!"

Don't tell Susan this, but helping someone to take off thirty-five pounds is one of our program's lesser miracles. Of course, that's not how Susan sees things. She finally got back to her size 9—easily! She's a youthful thirty-nine years old today. "Really, after so many years of trying and failing at programs, I had just about given up. Today, I see the bigger picture, which is that weight loss and good health are actually the same thing. And as I get older, that becomes really important to me."

BACK ON THE COURT

When Frank adopted our program, he was burdened with all the doubts you might expect from a man who hated the notion of "dieting," because he resisted the implicit suggestion that he was not only getting older, but also couldn't control his weight without a diet program. Also, Frank had already suffered enough on his own form of dieting, which essentially was a form of food deprivation. On top of all his other associations with dieting, he equated it with being hungry. In fact, he never would have adopted our program had it not been for his wife, who had read about the Pritikin approach in a magazine and bought one of my father's books.

When Frank and Marcie adopted the Pritikin Program, Frank was thirty pounds overweight; his blood cholesterol was 225 mg/dl, and his blood pressure was slightly elevated at 140 over 90. "I felt lousy," said Frank. "But I was in denial. I kept thinking that I would get the weight off eventually, and all my numbers would come back into the healthy ranges. But I never did anything about it, really. The few times I tried, I failed miserably. I hated dieting. And then Marcie and I went on the Pritikin Program. I've got to tell you, at first, I wasn't sure I could do it. It was a big change. But deep down inside, I really wanted to make a big change. Something inside me knew I had to do it, or I wouldn't ever get my life back. I'd just backslide forever till I died."

There were a couple of characteristics about our program that Frank liked a lot, however. "I liked the fact that I could eat all the time. I hated being hungry. Another thing—I always liked rice, and Marcie makes it with some lean chicken, vegetables, and mild spices, and I enjoy it. So now I'm eating lots of brown rice and other grains, lots of vegetables and fruits, and pretty soon I'm enjoying the food."

Frank was enjoying the results as well. He dropped thirty pounds in six months on the diet; his cholesterol level fell to 170 mg/dl, and his blood pressure normalized to 120 over 80. Though she was not significantly overweight to begin with, Marcie lost ten pounds, and her cholesterol level fell to 150 mg/dl. The biggest impact of the program has been on Frank. "I feel great," he said recently. "You know, once in a while I slip, but the fact is that on this program you don't really have to cheat in order to enjoy yourself. There are a lot of choices, a lot more than I originally thought."

One of the things that has really pleased Frank is that he's back on the court—this time the tennis court. "Yeah, we've got a few guys who play doubles. We're just hackers, but it's fun and we work up a sweat. Marcie and I get out and walk pretty religiously, too. We're out at least five days a week, and a couple of nights I play some tennis with the guys."

RENEE'S STORY

Renee, a thirty-six-year-old registered nurse from Michigan, was just over two hundred pounds when she began the Pritikin Program in March 1995. Not only was she overweight, but she felt terrible. "My knee joints ached, my back hurt. At age thirty-six, I moved like an old woman."

When she first began the program, Renee did not believe she could continue. "There's no way I'm going to be able to do this," she said upon starting it. The foods and their tastes were initially foreign to her. But she persevered for a few weeks, and in less than one month Renee had seen so many changes in her health and weight that she told her husband, "There is no way I'm not going to do this."

Renee was so committed to the Pritikin Program that she told her employers that she would have to start eating at her desk, which at that point was against office policy. After Renee explained what she was trying to do, her manager changed the policy. "This is something I need to do," she told her employer. "When I need to eat, I eat."

She maintained the same spirit about exercise. "When the weather's good, I walk outdoors. When it's bad, I walk at the gym or at the mall. If I can't get out, I exercise in my living room."

In less than a year, Renee had lost seventy-five pounds and kept the weight off. Today, she's a perfect size 8—fit and energetic, and younger than she's been in years.

THE PRITIKIN PROGRAM FOR OUTSMARTING THE FAT INSTINCT

THE PRITIKIN EATING PLAN

Our lives are defined in large measure by the choices we make. What most of us do not realize is that when it comes to choosing our foods, we usually don't choose at all. Instead, we are driven by our fat instinct to eat certain foods that will satisfy our hunger for fat and calorie-rich foods. As anyone who's ever been in the grip of a craving for fatty or calorie-rich foods knows, there's very little room for choice under such circumstances. The "choices" are either made unconsciously or spring from a need so strong that it borders on compulsion. Once the fat instinct is in full throttle, it's as if you're possessed. At that point, you really don't have much choice in the matter. You eat the foods you're craving.

Outsmarting your fat instinct and making food choices that will promote your health, optimal weight, and vitality is an act of self-empowerment. You are, in effect, taking back your power to make choices instead of succumbing to unconscious needs or urges. The effects of these healthier choices are significant and accumulate over time. One day, you wake up and find that you're lean, clear-eyed, energetic, and youthful looking. It didn't happen by accident, but is the effect of positive choices made consistently.

When you look over the Pritikin Eating Plan, you will see that there are a lot more choices on our program than you might have guessed. In fact, there isn't one situation that you might find yourself in—from being in a French restaurant to just wanting a snack while on the road—that our nutritionists and dietitians haven't accounted for, and provided you with a healthier choice. As you make those choices day after day, week after week, month after month, the effects will transform your life. In a very short time, people on the Pritikin Program experience a significant improvement in weight, vitality, and clarity of mind. Many feel more optimistic and positive about themselves and the future. The vast majority of people with high cholesterol levels see their cholesterols fall into the healthy ranges. Immune systems become stronger. The chances of contracting a serious disease, such as heart disease, cancer, adult-onset diabetes, or high blood pressure, decrease dramatically. All of these effects radically and positively transform people's lives.

STEPPING YOUR WAY TO HEALTH

Below you will find three sets of food choices under the headings "Better," "Better Still," and "Best," and as their titles suggest, each one represents a successive improvement in quality over its predecessor. If you are currently on the typical American diet, the foods listed under Better are much more healthful than the ones you are currently eating. Better represents the first step in an improved diet. The selections under Better Still are an improvement over Better, while Best represents the very highest-quality food choices, and the ones that provide people with the greatest opportunity to restore their health. All three sets of choices fall under the Pritikin Stepping Plan. They differ in their relative capacity to create fullness per calorie and their effects on your weight and health.

Below you will find seven days' worth of meal plans. For every breakfast, lunch, and dinner, there are Better, Better Still, and Best choices. We have done the same for snacks, as well as for fast foods and restaurant meals. No matter what situation you find yourself in, you can make a healthier choice, one that will provide the benefits of the Pritikin Eating Plan.

How to Make Good Eating Choices

There are two ways to approach the three sets of choices. The first is to see all three as a single diet in which you move from one set of choices to the next, even within the same day, depending on your circumstances and what you may want to eat at any given meal. For example, you may start out your day, as I do, with one of the Best breakfasts, such as oatmeal with cinnamon and herbal tea.

At around 10 A.M., you're ready for a snack, which, if you work at an office, you can eat at your desk. This morning, all you can manage is a low-fat bran muffin (a Better choice).

Later in the day, you have a business lunch and find yourself in a restaurant where your choices are limited and the best you can manage is a Better Still choice of a turkey breast sandwich (3½ ounces of turkey) on sourdough with mustard, lettuce, and tomato; a cup of salad with reduced-fat dressing; and a diet soda. It's certainly a healthful choice given the circumstances.

Now it's 2:30 or 3:00 P.M. and you find yourself getting a little hungry so you open a can of fruit packed in juice (a Best choice); or you take some hot water from the teapot or water cooler in the office and pour it into a ready-to-eat, dehydrated, fat-free, low-sodium cup of soup (also a Best choice). You eat your snack at your desk, along with a cup of tea.

You're tired by dinnertime and don't feel like cooking a lot of food, so you make 1½ cups of white pasta with primavera sauce. You sprinkle on one tablespoon of Parmesan cheese. You have a cup of salad with some low-fat dressing, a piece of sourdough bread, and a glass of dry wine. After dinner, you enjoy some sorbet. The whole meal takes you anywhere from twenty-five to thirty minutes to prepare and it's one of the Better dinners.

Later in the evening, you feel like a snack and a cup of tea, so you have some fat-free cookies (Better), or dried fruit (Better Still), or baked chips and bean dip (Best). If you want something savory, you can also have a bowl of soup (also a Best choice).

You've just spent a day on the Pritikin Eating Plan, moving up and down the Better, Better Still, and Best scale. You have not deviated once from the program. It's been a good day.

This is how I maintain the program in my own life. I try to make the best choice I can, depending on how I feel and the circumstances in which I find myself. For my own program, I try to stay as much as possible in the Best range, but it's not always possible. Sometimes, the best that's available is a Better choice and sometimes, I must admit, I flip right off the chart. But the next day, I'm up exercising, eating well, and back on the program. Occasional slips are going to happen, but with the kind of flexibility the Pritikin Eating Plan provides, it's easy to maintain consistency, especially after you have begun exercising and adapted your taste buds to these healthier foods.

A second way to use the Better, Better Still, and Best program is to choose one of the three levels and stay within that level consistently. In order to determine which of the three sets of choices you should adopt, you must first clarify the goals you want to achieve with the program, and then decide how you can best realize those goals.

The first and most important goal is your health, which of course includes your weight. When my father developed the program, there was essentially only one choice: a diet composed of 75 percent carbohydrates, 10 percent fat, 15 percent protein, and very low sodium. That's still the ideal Pritikin Program and the one that you will follow if you adopt the Best Pritikin choices and stick to them exclusively. The Best choices will result in the fastest and most dramatic improvements in health and weight.

I provide additional recommendations in the appendix for those concerned with specific illnesses, such as heart disease and high blood pressure. I also offer guidelines for people who are losing more weight on the program than they are comfortable with. (A certain minority of people find this to be a problem.)

You cannot consider your health goals, however, without also considering the kind of program you can maintain consistently. If you rigidly adopt the Best choices, but have trouble staying within that level, you may find yourself giving up on the program entirely. Consistency is the key to getting results. But consistency depends on what you can do. Don't establish goals you can't keep. That means that a lot of people should start out on the Better choices and work their way up to the Better Still and Best, as they incorporate the overall program into their lives. Start with what you can do, maintain that program every day, and move up as you become more adept and look to achieve better results.

It's important to realize that the Pritikin Program is not a prescription, but an approach to a healthy life. We've built tremendous flexibility and creativity into this program. We don't want you to feel as if you're in some kind of straitjacket. Just the opposite: We want you to feel that no matter what the circumstances, you can choose foods that you enjoy and, at the same time, promote your health. One of the keys to consistency, therefore, is being able to enjoy your food every day.

The irony is that the enjoyment you experience on this diet over time depends in part on your ability to maintain it. Consistency is the fastest and most efficient way to change your palate. Someone who follows a daily regimen of the type I described above will enjoy the food a lot sooner than someone who has sausage and eggs for breakfast, some vegetables for lunch, and steak for dinner. Not only will the latter person not experience any health improvement from such choices, but that vegetable lunch will be the least enjoyable meal of the day.

As we saw in chapter 6, our ancestors adapted their palates to the foods that nature provided. Such adaptation was essential to their survival, because enjoying the foods that were available kept them from searching for foods that weren't. They adapted their palates because their limited choices forced them to be consistent, which of course is not the case today. However, research has shown that when people maintain their low-fat diets consistently, they enjoy those diets just as much as their old regimens, and do not feel deprived of their high-fat foods.

Assisting your efforts at transforming your palate and enjoying the Pritikin Eating Plan are the five fundamental behaviors of the program:

1. Exercise, which increases your craving for high-carbohydrate foods, and also improves your health and helps to lower your weight

2. Choosing the right carbohydrate-rich food, which enables you to lose weight without hunger

3. Limiting your fat intake, which keeps your fat instinct dormant and your calorie intake low, and promotes health and weight loss

4. Eating frequently, which keeps you from being hungry, prevents the triggering of your fat instinct, and keeps your body burning fat

5. Maintaining consistency over time, which changes your palate and turns the program into a way of life

These five behaviors are the most important principles of the Pritikin Program. Combining them enables you to enjoy and even prefer the foods that will promote your health. When that happens, good health is the natural result of following your cravings and taste buds.

Part of being able to maintain these behaviors is knowing how to make healthful choices in the supermarket, at restaurants, or while traveling. The guidelines below will help you make food choices that are consistent with the five principles of the Pritikin Program.

GUIDELINES FOR MAKING HEALTHY CHOICES

Making the best food choice can sometimes be difficult, especially if you are in a situation in which your choices are limited. So here's a simple way to make the best choice in virtually any eating situation: *Choose foods that will provide you with the greatest sense of fullness on the fewest number of calories.*

Not surprisingly, the foods that will fill you up on the fewest calories, or those with the highest satiety value, are usually the ones that have the greatest positive impact on your health. You can assess the satiety value and healthfulness of any food, including those within the three categories of the Pritikin Eating Plan, by using four simple criteria:

1. How much fat does the food contain? Fat has low satiety value, which means that the more fat in a food, the more you will eat of that food before you feel full, or satisfied. Fat also contains the greatest concentration of calories. Fat will stimulate your fat instinct, so your chances of overeating that food will increase. Fat

not only increases your body fat and weight, but also impairs your health, increasing your chances of contracting heart disease, cancer, type II or adult-onset diabetes, and high blood pressure.

Thus, a simple rule of thumb: *Choose low-fat foods.*

2. How much fiber does the food contain? The more fiber in a food, the more filling it will be on the fewest number of calories. Plant foods, of course, are the source of fiber in the diet. They are also extremely low in calories, as I showed in chapter 4. Fibrous foods also slow absorption of sugars, which means they maintain your fat burning at relatively high levels. Thus, they contribute to weight loss.

   The simple guideline: *Choose the food with the most fiber.*

3. How much water does the food contain? Foods that contain water or are cooked in water—such as fresh vegetables, fruits, and cooked grains—provide fewer calories bite for bite than processed foods that contain concentrated calories. The sugars in dry foods, such as bread or dried cereals, are much more concentrated and rapidly absorbed than the sugars in fresh vegetables, fruits, cooked grains, or even pasta.

   The simple guideline: *Choose the food that contains water, or is cooked in water, and is the least processed food available. If you choose a processed food, choose one low in fat.*

4. What is the relative amount of simple sugars a food contains? Foods that contain relatively higher amounts of simple sugars cause the bloodstream to be overwhelmed by sugar. This causes your body to reduce its fat burning in order to burn the excess sugar in your blood. The result is that the fat in your tissues will be retained. Simple sugars appear most abundantly in processed foods, which often contain fat.

   The simple guideline: *Choose the food with the least amount of simple sugars.*

Here's a simple way to apply the four guidelines to create a healthful Italian meal. First, choose a marinara sauce instead of a meat sauce for your pasta, thus reducing the amount of fat in the meal. You can reduce the fat even further by cooking the marinara sauce without oil. Next, add vegetables to the sauce to create a pasta primavera. This will increase both the fiber and the water content of the meal, making absorption of the sugars even slower. You can increase the fiber even further by preparing whole wheat noodles. Finally, use a marinara sauce that does not contain sugar.

You've eliminated the fat, increased the fiber, included water in the preparation, and reduced the sugar, all of which has made this a healthy choice.

These guidelines can be applied to virtually any meal in the same way. A burrito can be made healthier by requesting that the pinto or black beans be made without lard. You can go even further by requesting that no guacamole be added; that only nonfat sour cream or cheese be used; and that salsa and rice be added for flavor. Finally, use a corn instead of a flour tortilla. Corn tortillas contain no fat, unlike those made of flour, which are cooked in lard.

These four criteria describe the differences among the three steps of the Pritikin Eating Plan. When taken as a whole, the Better regimen contains more fat, less fiber, less water, and more simple sugars than the Better Still and Best regimens, which means that you will consume more calories on the Better regimen than you will on the Better Still and Best.

As you progress from Better, to Better Still, to Best, the foods become increasingly satiating, or provide a greater sense of fullness per calorie. Therefore, the foods in the Better Still category will cause faster and more pronounced weight loss than those in the Better group, while the foods in the Best category will cause the most dramatic weight loss of all three categories. As you move from Better, to Better Still, to Best the regimens become increasingly health-promoting. The Best program is the most health-promoting program we can provide.

One of the impressive effects of fullness is that it immediately diminishes the influence of your fat instinct on your food choices. Fullness gives you a degree of freedom from the fat instinct so that you can make more healthful choices. Therefore, the foods in the Better Still and Best categories will have the greatest dampening effect on your fat instinct, and consequently provide you with the greatest degree of freedom from chronic hunger while you shed excess body fat.

Still, fullness is but one aspect of the larger experience that is part of being satisfied by your food. Satisfaction not only includes fullness, but also the pleasure we derive from the food's flavor. As far as I'm concerned, I want satisfaction from my food, and I'm sure you do, too.

Satisfaction has a lot to do with what you are craving at any particular moment, the kinds of foods you enjoy, and how hungry you are. All of these factors are highly flexible, and indeed they are subject to change over time, depending on what you grow accustomed to eating. If I planted you in northern Mexico among a tribe of native Americans called the Tarahumara, you'd be on a perfect diet because the Tarahumara eat foods almost exclusively from the Best Pritikin choices. After a while you'd adapt to that diet and you'd enjoy it. Pretty soon, you'd even find yourself craving foods that the Tarahumara crave.

You'd also be in excellent shape because the Tarahumara love to run. They play a game similar to soccer that requires the male participants to run more than one hundred miles without stopping. The women play the same game but run *only* sixty miles.

Not surprisingly, the Tarahumara enjoy what most of us would describe as excellent health. They experience virtually no heart disease, high blood pressure, cancer, type II or adult-onset diabetes, or other degenerative illnesses. They're lean and fit, by anyone's standards. If you lived among these people for a while, you'd change dramatically. Not only would you enjoy good health, optimal weight, tremendous fitness, and vitality, but you would also love the food, just as they do. How's that for a combination!

This is an illustration of how your environment can force you to be consistent. That consistency, in turn, will change your palate and alter what you think of as delicious and satisfying. This same effect occurs in people who move to another region of the country where the food is different, or to another country entirely, where the culture and cuisine are dramatically different from their own. For example, westerners who grew up eating steak, milk, and eggs, but later moved to Japan, often come to love the Japanese diet, including the sushi, rice, and vegetables. These same foods may have caused nausea back home, but they actually came to prefer the new foods over their old diets once they became accustomed to them.

Of course, it's unlikely that you're going to move to northern Mexico or Japan anytime soon, so you have to do the next best thing: practice the five principal behaviors on the Pritikin Program. Exercise regularly (this will create a craving for carbohydrate-rich foods); eat the right carbohydrates (this will create maximum satiety on the fewest calories); limit fat (this will keep the fat instinct at bay and promote optimal weight and health); eat frequently (you'll be full and burn more fat); and maintain consistency (which will rapidly retrain your palate).

These five behaviors are the keys to experiencing maximum satisfaction on the Pritikin Program. We have created a program with foods that are palatable, enjoyable, and satisfying. The more you practice the five Pritikin behaviors, the more palatable and enjoyable our diet becomes.

Don't forget that these same behaviors also give you some flexibility with your diet. After you start to incorporate our diet into your daily lifestyle, you'll see just how many delicious choices there are on the program already. Anyone can enjoy these foods immediately, but they become even more delicious and satisfying the longer you practice the program.

KNOW THE PROGRAM

One of the more effective television advertisements today is for V8 Juice, which includes the slogan, "I could have had a V8." The ad is very effective because it does two things: it reminds you in advance not to forget to have a V8 the next time you have a chance, and it suggests that the person in the commercial who is saying this now regrets the choices he made. You can almost feel his stomach ache, as he says, "I could have had a V8."

Try to learn and understand the Pritikin Eating Plan as quickly as you can so that you will be fully armed when you go into a high-quality or fast-food restaurant. By knowing the program, you will be able to choose well and be completely satisfied. I don't want you to walk out of that restaurant feeling sick and saying to yourself, "I could have had a Pritikin Better, Better Still, or Best meal."

Know the program so that you know your choices, no matter what situation you are in. That is the best way to maintain consistency and get results.

Eat Two Meatless Meals Per Day

The Best Pritikin Program recommends that you eat no more than $3\frac{1}{2}$ ounces of animal food per day, which is about the size of a deck of cards. In order to achieve this, we generally like to say that you should eat at least two meals per day composed entirely of plant foods. As you will see from the menu suggestions beginning on page 138, that's relatively easy to achieve.

THE PRITIKIN DIET: AN OVERVIEW

The Pritikin Eating Program is composed primarily of minimally processed plant foods loaded with carbohydrates in their natural state, low-fat animal foods, and an endless variety of spices, herbs, sauces, and dressings. The diet includes the following:

- A wide variety of leafy, stalk, and root vegetables, including asparagus, broccoli, brussels sprouts, carrots, celery, Chinese cabbage, collard greens, cucumber, endive, escarole, green beans, ginger, kale, leeks, lettuce, mushrooms, mustard greens, okra, onions, potato, radish, rutabaga, sweet potato, tomato, turnip, watercress, yams, and zucchini.

- Beans, including adzuki beans, black beans, black-eyed peas, chickpeas, great northern beans, kidney beans, lentils, lima beans, navy beans, pinto beans, and soybeans. Soy bean products, such as tofu and tempeh, are loaded with protective phytochemicals, including phytoestrogens.

- Fruits, such as apples, blackberries, blueberries, grapefruit, mangoes, oranges, papaya, pears, plums, and strawberries.

- Whole grains such as barley, brown rice, buckwheat, corn, millet, oats, rye, and wheat (including bulgur and whole wheat berries), as well as pasta.

- Low-fat animal foods (limited to 3 ¹/₂ ounces per day), including fish, the white meat of chicken and turkey, lean beef, egg whites, skim milk, and nonfat cheeses. The Best program allows one 3¹/₂-ounce serving of lean beef, fowl, or fish per day. It also includes 2 cups of skim milk, or two ³/₄-cup servings of nonfat yogurt, or 2 ounces of nonfat cheese, or ¹/₄ cup of nonfat cottage cheese.

- Herbs, spices, sauces and dressings (see recipes and menu suggestions).

This summary reflects the Best regimen, which provides maximum satiety on the fewest calories. It is loaded with vitamins and minerals that will boost your immune system and help prevent cancer, heart disease, stroke, and type II or adult-onset diabetes.

MENUS, SNACKS, FAST FOODS, AND RESTAURANT MEALS

This section contains menu plans for seven days; each day offers choices within the Better, Better Still, and Best categories. There are also snack ideas, suggestions for quality-restaurant eating and recommendations for meals at fast-food restaurants.

As you move up from Better to Best, you consume less fat and sugar and more fiber and water.

For example, one of the Better breakfasts includes 2 pancakes cooked in reduced-fat butter spray, syrup (2 to 3 tablespoons), 8 ounces of 1% milk, 6 ounces of fruit juice, and 1 cup of decaf. A Better Still Breakfast includes 1 cup of hot Cream of Wheat or grits, 8 ounces of 1% milk, 1 slice of whole-wheat toast, jam (1 tablespoon), ¹/₂ grapefruit, and 1 cup of decaf. One of the Best breakfasts includes 1¹/₃ cups hot oatmeal with cinnamon, 1 cup blueberries, 8 ounces of nonfat milk, and herbal tea.

Dinner has undergone a similar transformation. Among the Better dinner choices is 1½ cups chili con carne, 6 reduced-fat crackers, 1 cup salad with reduced-fat dressing, and a 12-ounce light beer. A Better Still choice includes chicken teriyaki rice bowl (2 ounces of chicken and 1½ cups of rice), 1 cup of salad with reduced-fat dressing, ½ cup of nonfat frozen yogurt, and iced tea or diet soda. Among the Best choices is 1½ cups of Vegetarian Chili, 1 baked potato, 1 cup of tomato and cucumber salad with balsamic vinegar, ½ cup of Pritikin Ice Cream, and mineral water. The more you use the three-step program, the quicker you will be able to design a Better, Better Still, and Best meal for yourself under just about any circumstance.

MENUS ✿ BREAKFAST

BETTER

Day 1
2 pancakes cooked in reduced-fat
    butter spray
Syrup (2 to 3 tablespoons)
8 oz. 1% milk
6 oz. fruit juice
1 cup decaf

Day 2
Egg-substitute omelet (equivalent of
    2 eggs) cooked in reduced-fat
    butter spray
2 slices Canadian bacon
1 slice raisin toast
4 oz. low-sodium V8 juice
1 cup decaf

Day 3
Low-fat bran muffin
Banana
6 oz. nonfat yogurt
1 cup decaf

Day 4
2 frozen low-fat waffles
Light maple syrup (2 tablespoons)
Sliced banana
1 cup decaf

Day 5
Egg-substitute omelet (equivalent of
    2 eggs) with fat-free cheese,
    cooked in reduced-fat butter
    spray
2 slices whole-wheat toast
2 tablespoons jam
1/3 cantaloupe
1 cup decaf

Day 6
3 blueberry pancakes cooked in
    reduced-fat butter spray
Light maple syrup (3 tablespoons)
8 oz. 1% milk
1 cup decaf

Day 7
2 oz. corn flakes or rice cereal or
    puffed rice
8 oz. 1% milk
6 oz. orange juice
1 slice whole wheat toast
Jam (2 tablespoons)
1 cup decaf

BETTER STILL

Day 1
English muffin with nonfat cream
    cheese or jam (2 tablespoons)

Banana
8 oz. 1% milk
1 cup decaf

Day 2
Egg-substitute omelet (equivalent of
  2 eggs) cooked in Pam
1 slice whole wheat toast
1 tablespoon fat-free cheese
Orange slices
1 cup decaf

Day 3
Bagel
1 slice fat-free cheese or fat-free
  cream cheese
Sliced tomato
Apple
1 cup decaf

Day 4
1 cup hot Cream of Wheat or grits
8 oz. 1% milk
1 slice whole-wheat toast
Jam (1 tablespoon)

1/2 grapefruit
1 cup decaf

Day 5
Hot "cereal in a cup" or instant
  oatmeal
2 tablespoons raisins
8 oz. 1% milk
1 cup decaf

Day 6
3 buckwheat pancakes
Apple butter (3 tablespoons)
Sliced banana
1 cup decaf latte (4 oz. nonfat milk)

Day 7
2 oz cold cereal (All-Bran, Cheerios)
8 oz. 1% milk
Sliced banana
6 oz. orange juice
1 cup decaf

BEST

Day 1
1 1/3 cups hot oatmeal with cinnamon
1 cup blueberries
8 oz. nonfat milk
Herbal tea

Day 2
Egg-substitute omelet (equivalent of
  2 eggs) with 1 1/2 cups of diced
  red potatoes and 1/2 diced onion,
  cooked in Pam
6 oz. nonfat yogurt
1 cup berries
Herbal tea

Day 3
1 1/3 cups hot Irish oatmeal or
  7-grain cereal
1 cup sliced peaches
8 oz. nonfat milk
Herbal tea

Day 4
1 1/3 cups hot multigrain cereal
Sliced banana
8 oz. nonfat milk
Fresh fruit cup
Herbal tea

Day 5
1 cup hot Wheatena
6 oz. nonfat yogurt
1 cup strawberries
Herbal tea

Day 6
3 oat bran–apple pancakes with
    diced apple and cinnamon

Sugar-free maple syrup
    (3 tablespoons)
½ grapefruit
Herbal tea

Day 7
1¼ cups shredded wheat with bran
8 oz. nonfat milk
1½ cups strawberries
Herbal tea

LUNCH

BETTER

Day 1
Roast beef on a French roll
1 cup salad with reduced-fat dressing
Iced tea or diet soda

Day 2
Bean and rice burrito with salsa and
    avocado slices (corn tortilla)
1 cup salad with reduced-fat dressing
Iced tea or diet soda

Day 3
Ham and cheese sandwich (97%
    fat-free ham and 1 slice nonfat
    cheese)
1 oz. reduced-fat potato chips
2 fat-free cookies
8 oz. 1% milk

Day 4
Cup of minestrone soup
Peanut butter and jelly sandwich
    (2 tablespoons natural peanut

butter, 2 tablespoons jam)
Applesauce
8 oz. 1% milk

Day 5
2 soft chicken tacos with lettuce
    and tomatoes (no sour cream,
    guacamole, or cheese)
Beans and rice
Iced tea or diet soda

Day 6
Stir-fried beef with broccoli
Steamed rice
Fortune cookie
Chinese tea

Day 7
Turkey subway sandwich on a roll
    (6-inch size) with mustard (no
    cheese or mayo)
1 oz. pretzels
6 oz. apple juice

BETTER STILL

Day 1
Grilled chicken sandwich (white bread, no mayo)
2 cups salad with reduced-fat or fat-free dressing
Diet soda

Day 2
Cup of hot and sour soup
Stir-fry vegetables (light on the oil) with 3 oz. shrimp or scallops
$1/2$ cup steamed rice
Chinese tea or mineral water

Day 3
Bagel
4 oz. sliced turkey breast
1% cottage cheese with sliced peach (fresh or canned in juice)
Trail mix
Diet soda

Day 4
Veggie burger on whole-wheat bun
1 slice nonfat cheese
2 cups salad with reduced-fat dressing
Hot tea or diet soda

Day 5
Cheeseless vegetarian pizza
2 cups salad with reduced-fat dressing
Diet soda

Day 6
Stir-fried vegetables with 3 oz. chicken
Steamed rice
Fortune cookie
Chinese tea

Day 7
Turkey breast (3 oz) sandwich on sourdough with mustard, lettuce, and tomato
1 cup salad with reduced-fat dressing
Diet soda

BEST

Day 1
Grilled chicken breast
Baked potato or corn on the cob
2 cups salad with fat-free dressing
1 cup steamed vegetables
Mineral water or herbal tea

Day 2
$1^{1}/_{2}$ cups whole-wheat pasta with
marinara sauce and steamed vegetables
2 cups salad with fat-free dressing or balsamic vinegar
Steamed asparagus spears
Mineral water or herbal tea

Day 3
Soup in a cup (dehydrated, fat-free)

1 cup raw vegetables
1/2 cup tuna salad with fat-free mayo in 1/2 whole-wheat pita bread
Apple or pear

Day 4
Pritikin 3-bean chili (1/2 can)
Baked potato
1 cup steamed frozen mixed vegetables
Orange
Decaf iced tea or sugar-free lemonade

Day 5
4 oz. broiled fish
Baked potato with 2 tablespoons nonfat sour cream

2 cups salad with fat-free dressing
1 cup fresh fruit salad (or canned packed in juice)
Mineral water

Day 6
2 oz. sashimi with wasabi and lemon
1 cup steamed vegetables
1 cup brown rice
Herbal tea or mineral water

Day 7
Turkey breast (2 oz.) sandwich on whole-wheat bread with mustard, lettuce, and tomato
1 cup vegetable soup
Apple or pear

DINNER

BETTER

Day 1
1 1/2 cups chili con carne
6 reduced-fat crackers
1 cup salad with reduced-fat dressing
12 oz. light beer

Day 2
1 1/2 cups white pasta with primavera sauce
1 tablespoon Parmesan
1 cup salad with reduced-fat dressing
1 slice sourdough bread
1/2 cup Italian ice
1 glass dry wine

Day 3
1 cup Chicken Curry*
1 cup white rice
1 cup salad with reduced-fat dressing
2 fat-free cookies
4 oz. nonfat frozen yogurt
Hot tea

Day 4
1 1/2 cups white linguine with quick clam sauce (bottled marinara, 3 oz.-can minced clams drained, 1 tablespoon oil)
1 cup salad with reduced-fat dressing

1 slice sourdough bread
4 oz. sorbet
1 glass dry wine

Day 5

1 1/2 cups beef and vegetable stew
(prepared with lean top sirloin)
1 bread or kaiser roll
1 cup salad with reduced-fat
dressing
1 slice fat-free cake
1 cup decaf

Day 6

1 1/2 cups couscous with 1 cup
grilled chicken and vegetables
1 small pita
2 fat-free cookies
1 cup decaf

Day 7

Pork tenderloin and vegetable stir-
fry (3 oz. pork, 2 cups vegetables)
1 cup white rice
1/2 cup orange sherbet
Hot tea

BETTER STILL

Day 1

1 1/2 cups Turkey Chili*
Whole-wheat roll
1 cup lettuce and tomato salad with
reduced-fat dressing
Iced tea or diet soda

Day 2

Chicken teriyaki rice bowl (2 oz.
chicken, 1 1/2 cups rice)
1 cup salad with reduced-fat
dressing
1/2 cup nonfat frozen yogurt
Iced tea or diet soda

Day 3

1 cup Chicken Curry*
1 cup brown rice
1 cup salad with reduced-fat
dressing
1/2 cup fat-free pudding
Hot tea

Day 4

1 1/2 cups white linguine with quick
clam sauce (no oil)
1 cup salad with reduced-fat
dressing
1/2 cup applesauce
Diet soda

Day 5

1 1/2 cups Belgian Chicken Stew*
Corn on the cob
1 cup salad with reduced-fat dressing
1/2 cup nonfat frozen yogurt
Diet soda

Day 6

1 1/2 cups couscous with 2 cups
grilled vegetables
1 small whole-wheat pita
1 cup salad with reduced-fat
dressing
Diet soda

Day 7
Chicken and vegetable stir-fry (2 oz. chicken, 2 cups vegetables)

1 cup white rice
1/2 cup fat-free, sugar-free pudding
Hot tea

BEST

Day 1
1 1/2 cups Vegetarian Chili*
1 baked potato
1 cup tomato and cucumber salad with balsamic vinegar
1/2 cup Pritikin Ice Cream*
Mineral water

Day 2
4 oz. poached salmon or boiled lobster with lemon
4 to 5 roasted new potatoes
1/2 cup asparagus
2 cups salad with balsamic vinegar
1/2 cup fruit salad
Hot herbal tea

Day 3
2 cups Red Pepper Lentil Stew*
2 cups salad with fat-free dressing
1/2 cup Pritikin Ice Cream*
Hot herbal tea

Day 4
1 1/2 cups whole-wheat pasta with quick clam sauce (no oil)

2 cups salad with fat-free dressing
1/2 cup strawberries
Mineral water

Day 5
2 cups Harvest Vegetable Stew*
2 cups salad with fat-free dressing
Fresh peach or pear
Hot herbal tea

Day 6
2 cups Bulgur Pilaf*
1 cup broccoli
2 cups salad with fat-free dressing
1/2 cup Chocolate Mousse*
Hot herbal tea

Day 7
1 cup vegetable soup
2 cups tofu veggie stir-fry (3 oz. tofu)
1 cup brown rice
1 orange
Hot herbal tea

SNACKS

This list of Pritikin-recommended snacks is also categorized Better, Better Still, and Best.

*See the recipe section.

BETTER

at-free tortilla chips
rail mix (no coconut)
.educed-fat or fat-free baked
  potato chips
efined fat-free muffins
.efined fat-free cookies

Refined fat-free crackers
Fat-free cheese
Peanut butter (drain oil)
Bagels
Pretzels
Soft pretzels (no butter)

BETTER STILL

Vhole-grain bagels
Vhole-grain fat-free muffins
Vhole-grain fat-free crackers
Vhole-grain fat-free cookies
at-free popcorn (no salt)
at-free pudding
)ried fruit

Fat-free fruit smoothie
Fat-free sugar-free yogurt
Fat-free sugar-free pudding
Sugar-free Jell-O
Fat-free sugar-free cocoa
Low-sodium V8

BEST

Raw veggies (fresh or prepackaged)
at-free low-sodium soups
  (dehydrated or canned)
Baked sweet potatoes
Baked or steamed red potatoes
Fresh fruit

Easy-open canned fruit, packed in
  juice
Bean dip
Salsa
Applesauce, unsweetened

RESTAURANT MEALS

Going out to restaurants and remaining on the Pritikin Program is a lot
easier than you may think. We have provided recommendations for several kinds of restaurants, including Mexican, Italian, Chinese, Japanese,
French, and American. Look over the choices carefully, commit them to
memory, and follow the recommendations. You'll have no trouble getting a Pritikin meal at the vast majority of good-quality restaurants.

MEXICAN

BETTER

Steamed corn tortillas
Salsa
Green salad, oil and vinegar
  dressing

Black bean burrito (with oil, no lard)
  sliced avocados, green chili sauce
Mexican rice
1 light beer

BETTER STILL

Steamed corn tortillas
Salsa
Green salad, oil and vinegar
  dressing

Chicken enchilada with salsa (no cheese)
Chicken fajitas
Mexican rice
Mineral water or decaf

BEST

Steamed corn tortillas
Salsa
Black bean soup

Soft tacos with chicken, lettuce, and
  tomato (no cheese)
Mineral water or herb tea (bring
  your own)

ITALIAN

BETTER

Antipasto of marinated artichoke
  hearts, mushrooms, peppers, etc.
Green salad, oil and vinegar dressing
Linguine with clam sauce

1 tablespoon Parmesan cheese
Italian or sourdough bread
Italian ice or sorbet with fresh fruit
1 glass of wine

BETTER STILL

Mussels Marinara

Green salad, oil and vinegar dressing

Linguine alla checca (tomatoes, basil, garlic, olive oil)
1 tablespoon Parmesan cheese
Italian or sourdough bread

Fresh fruit
Decaf cappuccino with nonfat milk

BEST

Minestrone soup
Salad with fat-free dressing or balsamic vinegar
Pasta with marinara sauce
Fish (grilled dry or poached)

Side order of steamed vegetables
Bread roll (sourdough or whole wheat)
Fresh berries
Mineral water

CHINESE

BETTER

Moo-shu vegetables (thin pancake with vegetables and hoisin sauce)
Stir-fry chicken and snow peas (easy on the oil and soy sauce)

Stir-fried vegetables (easy on the oil)
Steamed rice
1 light beer

BETTER STILL

Chinese noodles in broth
Stir-fry chicken and vegetables (easy on the oil and soy sauce)

Steamed vegetables
Steamed rice
Chinese tea

BEST

Steamed or baked whole fish with ginger and garlic (don't eat skin)
Stir-fried vegetables (no fat, use wine) or

Steamed vegetables
Steamed rice
Mineral water or herb tea (bring your own)

JAPANESE

BETTER

Maki sushi (raw tuna and seaweed)
Chicken teriyaki
Stir-fried vegetables

Steamed rice
1 beer

BETTER STILL

Oshinko (pickled vegetables)
Chicken sukiyaki
Steamed rice

Fresh fruit plate
1 light beer

BEST

Edamame (steamed green soy
  beans)
Miso soup
Tossed salad with miso dressing

Tuna sashimi
Steamed rice
Tea or mineral water

FRENCH

BETTER

Soup du jour (no cream)
House salad (dressing on the side)
Filet mignon (wine sauce on the
  side)

Vegetables du jour (no butter)
1 glass of wine

BETTER STILL

Baby green salad (dressing on the
  side)
Steamed mussels

Grilled vegetables
Fresh raspberries and fruit sorbet
Decaf and mineral water

BEST

Baby green salad (with balsamic vinegar or dressing on the side)	Boiled new potatoes and asparagus
Poached salmon	Fresh strawberries
	Herb tea and mineral water

AMERICAN

BETTER

Green salad (dressing on the side; use sparingly)	Baked potato
	Low-fat frozen yogurt
Bowl of chili con carne (no cheese)	1 glass wine and decaf

BETTER STILL

Vegetable soup	Baked potato
Grilled chicken breast	Sorbet
Steamed vegetables	Light beer and decaf

BEST

Large salad with balsamic vinegar	Baked potato
Broiled fish (no oil if possible)	Fresh fruit
Steamed vegetables	Herb tea (bring your own)

HEALTHY FAST FOOD

The cuisine turned out by fast-food restaurants is not what comes to mind when you think of the Pritikin Eating Plan, but you might be surprised that even in these proverbial dens of iniquity, you can remain on the program. There are so many choices within the fast-food industry that perhaps we're finally having an impact on their menus. You can help change these restaurants even more rapidly by ordering healthfully. If more and more of us demand healthful meals in fast-food restaurants, they will have to change to meet a growing demand for healthful fare.

BETTER

Cheeseless vegetable pizza
  Found at: Most pizzerias on request
Roast beef sandwiches (mustard, lettuce, tomato, whole wheat bread if possible, no mayo)
  Found at: Arby's
Rotisserie chicken (white meat only; remove the skin)

Found at: Boston Market, El Pollo Loco, Koo Koo Roo
Grilled/roasted chicken pita
  Found at: Jack in the Box
BBQ chicken sandwich (mustard, tomato, lettuce, whole wheat bread if possible, no mayo)
  Found at: Carl's, Jr.

BETTER STILL

Turkey breast sandwich (mustard, lettuce, tomato, whole wheat bread if possible, no mayo)
  Found at: All delis, Koo Koo Roo, Subway
Vegetable sandwich (mustard, no mayo)
  Found at: Subway, delis upon request
Charbroiled or grilled chicken breast sandwich (no mayo)

Found at: Boston Market, Wendy's, Chic-fil-A, Dairy Queen, Hardee's, Carl's, Jr.
Roast potatoes
  Found At: Sizzler, Boston Market, Kenny Rogers
Baked beans
  Found at: Kentucky Fried Chicken, El Pollo Loco, Boston Market, Kenny Rogers

BEST

Garden salads (fat-free dressing or no dressing)
  Found at: Wendy's, Hardee's, Arby's, Subway, McDonald's, Boston Market, Sizzler
Corn on the cob (no butter)

Found at: El Pollo Loco, Kentucky Fried Chicken, Boston Market, Kenny Rogers
Baked potatoes (no toppings)
  Found at: Sizzler, Wendy's, Carl's, Jr.

Steamed vegetables
  Found at: Boston Market, Koo
  Koo Roo, Sizzler, Kenny Rogers
Fresh fruit

Found at: Boston Market, Koo
Koo Roo, Sizzler, Kenny Rogers

FOUNDATION FOR YOUR HEALTH

In order to maintain the Pritikin Program and make healthful choices wherever you are, all you have to remember are five things: Exercise daily; eat the carbohydrate that is closest to its natural form; limit fat intake; eat frequently; and maintain consistency. As you incorporate the program into your life, you will naturally become familiar with all the food choices available to you, both at home and in restaurants.

As you come to know the satiety value of individual foods, choose the food that will fill you up on the least number of calories. Satiety value is determined by the amount of fat, fiber, water, and simple sugars in the food.

As you become adept at making healthful choices in all kinds of situations, you'll be able to forget that you're even on a program. You'll make healthy choices without ever feeling restricted, or even having to think very much about it. At that point, your daily life is the foundation for your health. Optimal weight and great vitality will be yours.

TRIGGERS AND THE NET

You're walking in a shopping mall, innocent of all other appetites except the singular intention of buying yourself a new shirt or blouse, when suddenly your nostrils are filled with the smell of chocolate chip cookies being baked by a nearby vendor. Forget the shirt or blouse. You want a cookie, or maybe several cookies, or maybe a whole bag of them. Or you arrive at a party and your host has laid out a spread of high-fat delicacies and alcoholic beverages that's downright bacchanalian. You were hungry when you showed up and now you're starved. All you can think about is which ten things you should eat first. Or you've had a rough day at the office, nothing went right, you're late on a deadline, and everyone is blaming you for the trouble. The day ends and you head home, feeling defeated. You're eager to take off your shoes, sit down before a big meal, and drown your miseries in food and drink.

Sound familiar? It's real life—or at least the part of life dominated by the fat instinct. Certain kinds of situations have a unique power to rouse the fat instinct from its dormant state within us and bring it forth with all its fury. Suddenly, you're in its grip, possessed by an overpowering urge to eat high-fat, high-calorie foods and drinks. Once the fat instinct has control of you, it's virtually impossible to discipline yourself from eating, or rather overeating. The most common result is weight gain or a setback to your health. I call these situations "triggers" because they elicit, or trigger, the fat instinct. The situations I cited above are three examples of very ordinary triggers. In fact, there is an endless array of triggers, most of which we all share, but some are unique to each of us.

Your fat instinct is being stimulated constantly by these trigger situations and events. Unfortunately, you're probably not aware of half of them. There are numerous strategies you can use to satisfy your hunger so thoroughly that you can release yourself from your fat instinct's grip. In this chapter, I want to share with you some of the ways I control my fat instinct, and especially how I deal with trigger situations every day. By doing that, I hope to give you some ideas on how you can incorporate the Pritikin Program into your daily life, and thereby protect yourself from the influences of the fat instinct.

I refer to the strategies that keep the fat instinct at bay as your "safety net," or simply "the net." The net can catch you from falling off the program entirely. It protects you when you are feeling weak or vulnerable to the influences of the fat instinct, which is the undoing of every diet and health program yet invented.

The primary strands of the net, of course, are the five principle behaviors that form the foundation of the Pritikin Program, as outlined in chapter 6. But, in addition, there are several steps you can take to keep yourself free of the fat instinct's influence. In order to realize your health and weight goals, you have to create your own net, or a support system that helps you maintain your health. Here are some of the things I do each day to keep the fat instinct at bay.

STRATEGY #1: CHOOSE THE ACTIVITY THAT YOU WILL MAINTAIN

The two most important behaviors that keep me beyond the reach of the fat instinct each day are exercise and avoiding hunger, and of these two, I would have to say that exercise is the single most important deterrent to the fat instinct. Before you jump to any conclusions, you must first understand what I mean by exercise, and why it's important. By exercise, I simply mean walking—and sometimes even short walks or strolls.

The American College of Sports Medicine (ACSM)—the most authoritative body of scientific experts on the subject of exercise—offers two sets of guidelines, one referred to as "ACSM light," and the other as "ACSM regular" or "traditional." If you are not currently exercising, I recommend you start out on ACSM light, which urges you to get thirty minutes or more of "moderately intense" physical activity most days of the week, and preferably every day. Two miles of walking per day at a comfortable pace meets that recommendation beautifully.

What most people do not realize is that the ACSM recommendation is based on *accumulated* minutes, which means that you can do ten minutes in the morning, ten minutes in the afternoon, and ten minutes in the evening to get your thirty minutes of walking in each day. The pace at which you walk does not have to be fast, or power walking, but moderate. Even strolling is sufficient, provided you walk long enough. Distance is more important than how fast you walk.

A primary reason we want you to exercise on the Pritikin Program is that it depletes your carbohydrate storage tanks in your muscles, keeps your fat burning high, and makes you crave carbohydrate-rich foods. As you exercise more and more, the Pritikin diet will seem like the most natural way to eat.

Doing the ACSM light begins to accomplish this goal. I encourage you to walk in the morning or the evening—whichever you most prefer and can maintain—and then walk throughout the day, whenever possible, even if it's just a short walk around the block at lunch. Be active—even in little ways, like short walks—throughout the day.

Of course, there are many other benefits to this amount of exercise. Walking is an aerobic exercise, meaning that it increases the flow of oxygen to muscles. Aerobic exercise strengthens the heart, lungs, large muscle groups, and bones. It can raise HDL levels, which reduces your risk of heart disease and stroke. And it lowers blood pressure. Studies have shown that moderate exercise boosts the immune system and protects against cancer. Exercise increases the body's demand for fuel and burns calories that are stored as fat. Thus, it reduces weight. Finally, studies have shown that exercise elevates mood significantly. It has even been shown to relieve chronic depression.

My father used to make a point of getting as much exercise as he could each day. He used to run three miles every morning, but he also took short runs and walks during the course of the day. I remember on many occasions when someone would come by unexpectedly to see him, he'd start the conversation while walking, or even running, to the street corner and back. It would only take a few minutes, but he was constantly finding ways of burning calories.

You can find hundreds of ways to get exercise through the course of the day, as well. Make a habit of taking the stairs to your office instead of the elevator, or take the elevator to a floor that is several stories below your office and then walk up the rest of the way. You can take a quick walk in the morning, at lunch, or in the afternoon. Before dinner, you can walk for ten or twenty minutes. After a very short while, you will begin to see yourself in a whole new light—as fit, lean, and active. Of course, all of this activity will have a tremendous impact on your diet and health, because the benefits you derive from exercise are cumulative, meaning the more exercise you do, the greater the benefits you derive.

You can satisfy the exercise part of the Pritikin Program and increase your desire for carbohydrate-rich foods simply by walking every day. And the more you do the better.

Do What Will Work for You

The question is, How can you ensure that you will walk every day? Each of us has to create a truly workable strategy to incorporate exercise into our lives. If we don't, exercise will be little more than a fantasy.

Before the participants in each of our program sessions graduate, we conduct a workshop where we ask people what their strategies will be to ensure that they will exercise every day, or at least four or five times per week. Invariably, the vast majority of them say that once they get home, they plan to start walking.

Good, we say. Where are you going to walk?

People respond with a variety of answers: In the park. Around the block. In the woods behind my house.

Okay, we say. But where do you live? More than sixty-five thousand people have participated in our programs at our centers in Santa Monica and Miami in the past twenty years and we get people from all over the country, and indeed all over the world. A great many of these people are from four-season climates, so when we ask the question

Where do you live? it's common to hear Minnesota, New York, Pennsylvania, Michigan, and many other places that have significant winters as answers.

Walking outdoors is great half the year, we say, but what are you going to do when it snows? Some are already walking year-round and have no trouble walking or cross-country skiing when the snow falls. Others look inward, confront their doubts, and then say, We'll walk in the shopping mall.

Okay. In fact, many will walk in the shopping mall—especially people who like to shop—but others find that walking in the mall eventually gets boring, and still others refuse to get near a mall for anything but the bare essentials. When we point this out, many answer by saying that they will join a health club.

That's a good idea, we say. Health clubs work. They provide wonderful facilities, including treadmills and weight-training equipment. Many have swimming pools and indoor racquetball and tennis courts. Also, some people join with a friend so that they do their workouts together. But then we ask, Have you ever joined a health club before? Many people answer, yes, they have been members of a health club, but they quit. In fact, many people have joined and quit health clubs lots of times. Why? One of the most common responses to that question is that the club's members were very different types of people from themselves.

The people who come to the Longevity Center are from all walks of life, but most of them are middle-aged or older people who are concerned about their health and their weight. They are not the kind of people who feel comfortable going to a club that caters to young men and women who want to lift weights, tone every muscle until it ripples, and stare at themselves in the mirror all day. So the next question we ask is this: Can you join a health club that is composed of people who are like you?

Yes, people answer. They know of such a club or they can find one.

That's good, we say, because a club that you feel comfortable joining is one you're likely to remain a member of.

But then we ask: Is the club within six to eight miles from your home, because if it's greater than ten miles from your house, you probably will end up quitting again. Studies have shown that when a health club is at a significant distance from one's house, it eventually becomes inconvenient to go there on a regular basis. In other words, people quit.

At that point, people begin to look baffled. What can we do? they ask. We want to exercise, but we have to make it work within our lives.

And that is exactly right. In order to ensure that you will get exercise every day, you have to create a strategy that works for you, and your unique circumstances. There is no universal answer, but there is an answer for everyone.

Here's What Works at the Longevity Center

Over the past twenty years, we have tried every conceivable motivation technique and piece of exercise equipment under the sun at the Longevity Center. Our long experience has taught us that treadmill machines are the single piece of equipment that people will use and continue using *for exercise*—rather than as a clothes hanger. New technology has provided treadmills with a flexible, shock-absorbing deck that can reduce the shock to the knees by as much as 30 percent. The soft surface that you walk on actually moves with you, so that there is no resistance against which you have to walk. This has the effect of supporting you as you exercise, moving you along. In effect, you must keep up with the treadmill, much the way you would if you were walking with a friend who was setting the pace. You can create a range of speeds and inclinations, as well, on a treadmill, so that you can start out slowly, increase speed after you've warmed up, and then slow and cool down as you complete your session.

Treadmills can be set up in front of a television set or by a stereo so that you can be entertained while you are on the machine. You don't even have to think about the fact that you are exercising while you watch TV or listen to music.

Treadmills are also extremely convenient. You can do ten, twenty, or thirty minutes of walking at any time of the day. For me, a treadmill is the basis of my daily exercise program. Indeed, breakfast and a session on the treadmill is how I start every day.

Pick a Time That's Good for You and Stick to It

Even though I encourage you to exercise throughout the day, I also think it's best to work out consistently at a particular time of the day. For the vast majority of us, the mornings are the best time to exercise, because most of us are most disciplined then. Studies have shown that those who exercise in the morning are most likely to be the ones still exercising a year later; those who exercise later in the day are the least likely to continue their exercise program.

I get up at between 6:30 and 7 A.M. and have some oatmeal (often I put some fruit in the oatmeal) and tea. Then I get on my treadmill and exercise for a half hour to forty minutes while I watch CNN's *Headline News*. This is a routine, a habit. I'm most in control of my environment and behavior in the morning, and consequently I'm able to get my day off to a good start.

As soon as I've finished my exercise and have showered, I eat a piece of fruit, usually in the car on the way to work. If I miss this small snack, my hunger increases and I experience a dip in energy. That's when I'm vulnerable to the fat instinct, so that piece of fruit on the way to work is important to me, which brings me to the second most important strategy for keeping the fat instinct at bay.

STRATEGY #2: AVOID HUNGER

The strongest trigger for the fat instinct, the one we all share, is hunger. If you allow yourself to get too hungry, you're most vulnerable to eating foods that contain fat or processed carbohydrates or both, which means you're most likely to eat foods that will cause weight gain. Hunger has a way of making you feel vulnerable and weak, as well. It triggers your survival instinct, which in turn summons the fat instinct from its lair.

The best tools for dealing with hunger are high-satiety, low-calorie foods, which we encourage you to eat frequently throughout the day. I use high-satiety foods as a protector against the fat instinct in every conceivable situation, from choosing snacks, to eating in restaurants, to traveling. Oatmeal for breakfast, for example, is a high-satiety, bulky food. It fills me up on relatively few calories. My fruit snack on the way to work is another good example of a low-calorie, high-satiety food.

After I've been at work for about an hour or so, I eat a snack, usually a cup of vegetable soup. This is especially common in the winter, when I tend to want to eat heavier meals and eat more frequently. The soup fills me up and gives me real satisfaction on very few calories. It also provides me with lots of energy so I'm well fortified for the morning.

I eat lunch at the Pritikin Longevity Center, except on days when I'm traveling or going out for a business lunch, so I have an advantage of getting good food most days of the year. But even when I travel or go out, I can still manage to get a good meal in virtually any restaurant, because the Pritikin strategy can be used anywhere.

One of the moments I'm most vulnerable to the fat instinct is when I walk into a restaurant and I'm hungry. The triggers are everywhere: The hunger conjures up images of big, rich meals, a few beers, and a big dessert when I'm done. My hunger is only exacerbated by the fact that I have to wait for a menu, and then to order, and then for the meal to arrive. The waiting, which sometimes seems interminable, tempts me to order foods that later on I might regret, simply because the fat instinct is compelling me to fortify myself with excess calories.

Okay, I'm hungry and I'm waiting and what does the waiter put in front of me: bread and butter, or bread and olive oil, or breadsticks that have been cooked in oil, or pizza bread. And then the waiter asks me if I want a drink. Triggers, triggers, and more triggers.

So here's what I do to outsmart the fat instinct. Even before I consider the menu, I order a high-satiety, low-calorie appetizer and have the waiter bring it to me right away. I always get a salad with a low-fat dressing "on the side." The salad alone takes the edge off my hunger and immediately dampens my fat instinct. If there's a good soup available, I'll get that, too. These two foods alone make me comfortable. Once I'm relatively sated, I can examine the menu. Whatever else I eat from that moment on, I do not feel compelled by my fat instinct to overeat or gorge. In other words, I can make wise choices.

From there, I choose the highest-satiety foods as main parts of my meal, which, of course, are the carbohydrate-rich vegetables, fruits, and grains. Pasta is often a good choice, as well, because it fills you up, but at the same time is slowly absorbed. You will recall from chapter 1 that fish is also a high-satiety food. It is very effective at filling you up, even on a relatively small portion of 3¹/₂ ounces.

At the Longevity Center, we follow the same strategy: we put the salad at the front end of the buffet so that people will fill up on highly nutritious, low-calorie vegetables. The lowest-satiety foods, such as the bread, are at the end of the food line. If you start out with a low-satiety food, you're going to eat a lot more of that food before you're satisfied, which means you're going to get a lot more calories than you really needed in order to feel full.

Making sure you have high-satiety, low-calorie foods available is one of the keys to healthy and enjoyable travel, as well.

Have Snacks, Will Travel

I'm especially vulnerable to the fat instinct when I travel or have a lot of meetings away from the office. A lot of people plan well when they travel, bringing all kinds of healthful foods, snacks, and soups to eat on the plane or at their hotel. They also order vegetarian or low-fat entrees from the airline. This, of course, is the right way to travel, and when I think to do such things I always congratulate myself. Unfortunately, I don't always do it. When I forget to bring snacks with me, or order a low-fat meal in advance, I usually buy something at one of the delis at the airport. A common choice is a turkey sandwich with lettuce and tomato, no mayonnaise, on whole-grain bread. I also get a soft pretzel, and bring both with me on the plane. The pretzel is a processed food that contains salt, but little or no fat. I brush off the salt and eat that as a snack on the plane. Often, I can get something on the plane that is decent, even if I have to eat around some of the more toxic fare. At the very least, there's a salad. If I don't feel like lemon as a dressing, I cheat a little by dipping my fork into the airline's vinaigrette dressing and then put the fork into the salad. That way, I get the taste of the dressing without loading it on the vegetables.

The first thing I do when I arrive at my hotel is order a big salad and a bowl of soup. I don't spend too much time with the menu—it gets me into trouble. Rather, I make a couple of quick healthy choices and then let it go. Once my stomach is full, I can think better and plan my schedule.

A very powerful trigger for me is alcohol before I order dinner. Restaurants sometimes encourage you to sit down and have a drink before you order, but that can be a disaster, because you can easily order a lot more food than you would have if you ate something satiating immediately upon entering. Not only does alcohol contain significant calories, but it encourages the fat instinct. People want high-calorie foods to nibble on when they drink, such as peanuts or cheese. There are enough calories in 8 ounces of peanuts to require half a marathon to burn off. The way I derail this track is by ordering some sparkling water and lime, along with my salad and soup. Like the salad and soup, sparkling water dampens a certain urge. If you're going to have a drink at dinner, don't order the wine until after you've ordered your meal.

STRATEGY #3: WHENEVER POSSIBLE, MAKE A PREEMPTIVE STRIKE

Recently, my wife, Christine, and I were in Miami where a festival was taking place that celebrated the many types of ethnic cuisines of the people who live in the city. Vendors standing behind their carts provided an endless supply of hamburgers and hot dogs; racks of lamb and beef, rotating on skewers; French fries crackling in hot oil; fried onions sizzling in huge frying pans; exotic dishes of rice, beans, and spices; barbecued chicken; and enough ice cream and cotton candy to last several lifetimes. The smells alone could make you crazy with the fat instinct. And not surprisingly, all the vendors were doing great business.

There are times when I feel I have to watch myself because if I ever start to indulge my fat instinct in the wrong place, someone might walk up to me and say, "Aren't you Robert Pritikin, son of Nathan—of the *low-fat diet* Pritikins?" In fact, that kind of thing has happened to me. Once, when I was in high school, my friends and I went to a Mexican restaurant where my friends proceeded to order every possible high-fat choice on the menu. I had ordered something innocuous, like a chicken enchilada on a corn tortilla, with salsa but no cheese. Unfortunately, their food came first and crowded the table, making it look like a smorgasbord of multicolored fat. Before my own food arrived, one of my high school teachers walked over to our table and said, "Robert Pritikin. What are you doing here?" I braced myself to be criticized, but my meal arrived in the nick of time. "Well, that looks very good," she said approvingly, and then left.

Still, recollections of such experiences tend to cross my mind before I indulge my temptations—and I must admit that the sting of such memories has kept me from making a lot of bad choices in public—but as Christine and I strolled through the Miami food fair, neither of us felt any real temptation to eat any of that food. The reason was simple: both of us had already eaten before we went to the festival. We had made what I like to call a "preemptive strike" against the fat instinct before we arrived, and so these trigger situations had been neutralized, as it were.

With my fat instinct dormant, I was free to wander throughout the festival and enjoy the sunny day, the friendly atmosphere, and the wonderful smells—and truly, these were smells worth lingering over—and not feel any compulsion to eat foods that, later on, I would be sorry I ever got near.

Essentially, making a preemptive strike means eating frequently. Eat whenever you are hungry, but think of yourself as needing three meals, plus three snacks per day in order to keep the fat instinct at bay.

This is especially important when you have to go out socially.

A major trigger for me is a party, banquet, or some other social engagement where high-fat foods and calorie-rich drinks are served. I get caught up in the socializing and the levity, and before I know it I'm eating unconsciously—or, rather, I'm eating according to the dictates of the fat instinct. Forget the use of discipline, at that point. I'm going to eat everything that's served—and make it a double.

But there's a key to these kinds of events that either makes me vulnerable to the fat instinct or frees me from its influences. That key is hunger. One of the worst things I can do to make myself vulnerable to the fat instinct is to go to such an affair hungry. Hunger is what the fat instinct needs to gain control over us. On the other hand, if I eat something before I go, I am free to enjoy myself and not feel compelled to overeat, especially on calorie-rich foods. Thus, every time I go to a social engagement, such as a party or a professional banquet, I eat something before going. I never go to a social engagement so hungry that I'm vulnerable to the fat instinct.

The same advice applies whenever you go grocery shopping: Don't go to a store hungry, because you will bring home all kinds of high-fat, high-calorie foods. It will be the fat instinct that's doing the shopping, not your rational self.

STRATEGY #4: MAKE YOUR ENVIRONMENT SUPPORT YOUR HEALTH

I believe that most of us are attracted to like-minded people who are sensitive to the same issues we are. In many ways, you and your friends reinforce each other on all kinds of beliefs that you have in common.

Not only do people influence each other's behaviors, but they also tend to benefit or suffer from the consequences of those behaviors. Hence, if you are conscious of your eating and exercise patterns, chances are that your friends will be too—and all of you will be healthier for it.

I do not preach the Pritikin Program to my friends. When I go out to dinner with friends, I want to put my work aside and just enjoy myself. I do not want to put pressure on anyone to be different; nor do I want to call attention to my own lifestyle. Still, I order my meals the same way I always do, and despite the fact that I am being as understated as possible, such behavior influences the people around me in a quiet way, especially over time. I have had the same core group of friends for many years, and they have become more like me than I have become like them, at least as far as their health habits are concerned. Today, these friends eat essentially healthy diets and are active, even without my having to make an effort to change their

behavior. And in many ways, we reinforce that behavior among ourselves and thereby enjoy the benefits.

A good example of this is a twelve-year follow-up study published
in *The British Medical Journal* (June 25, 1994) in which scientists
examined the death rates from heart disease and cancer among vegetarians and their meat-eating friends and relatives. As expected, the
vegetarians had significantly lower heart disease and cancer death
rates than the general population. What was surprising, however, was
that the friends and relatives of the vegetarians also had a much lower
risk of dying of cancer and heart disease than the general population,
even though these friends and relatives ate meat. Vegetarians had
only 28 percent of the risk of dying of heart disease that the general
population had, and only half the risk of dying of cancer. Remarkably,
their meat-eating friends and relatives also had less of a risk of dying
of both diseases—a 50 percent less risk of dying of heart disease and a
20 percent less risk of dying of cancer. Thus, both the vegetarians and
their friends and relatives were a lot less at risk of getting these diseases than the average person on the street was. What I always say
when I tell people about this study is that you don't have to be a vegetarian to enjoy the health benefits of a meatless diet—just be a friend
of a vegetarian!

The friends of vegetarians don't have improved health and reduced
risk factors simply because they know a vegetarian, of course. They
have less disease because their behaviors are influenced by their vegetarian friends. When they accompany their vegetarian friend to a
restaurant, they're likely to avoid a high-fat meal. They probably
realize that a high-fat diet is no good for them in the first place, and
since their vegetarian friend is making wiser choices, they might as
well, too.

Two or three days a week, I work out on the weight-training equipment at the center. The whole routine only takes about thirty minutes, but some days I'm about as eager to do that workout as I am to
take an ice-cold shower. Fortunately, I arrange in advance to do the
workout with a friend, sometimes two friends. We keep each other
going. My friends experience just as many days of resistance to exercise as I do, but fortunately for all of us, it's rare that our resistance to
exercise falls on the same day. Consequently, when I'm feeling lazy,

one of my friends is usually raring to go, just as when one of them doesn't feel like exercising, I'm eager for a workout. In this way, we keep each other in shape.

Weight or resistance training is worth considering for everyone, even if you're well into your nineties. Like aerobic exercise, weight training can raise HDL levels, lower blood pressure, and build stronger muscles and bones. Resistance training makes muscles larger, which means they become bigger tanks for carbohydrate storage. That larger carbohydrate storage capacity helps to keep your blood sugar levels lower, which means you burn more fat.

Unfortunately, the reverse is also true: People who live under the constant pull of the fat instinct can easily influence their friends to do the same, which in a relatively short time has deleterious effects on health. This can happen to people who are on the very best diet and exercise program, but suddenly fall under the control of the fat instinct. The Tarahumara Indians learned the power of the fat instinct firsthand.

In chapter 7, I mentioned the Tarahumara Indians of Mexico, who eat a diet extremely low in fat and who enjoy incredible fitness, due in part to a game they play during which the men run approximately one hundred miles. As I reported, the Tarahumara have extremely low rates of heart disease. They have low blood cholesterol levels and they are lean. In 1991 longtime diet and health researcher William Connor, his wife, Sonja (also a researcher and dietitian), and their colleagues found it quite easy to get the Tarahumara Indians to eat a high-fat, high-cholesterol diet typical of affluent societies. After eating this diet for only five weeks, the average blood cholesterol level among the Tarahumara increased 31 percent (from 121 mg/dl to 151 mg/dl) and they gained more than eight pounds. The Tarahumara live on the best diet and exercise program under the sun, and have lived that way for perhaps thousands of years. Yet, even they are not immune from the fat instinct. And once they started eating according to the dictates of the fat instinct, it would have been hard for them to stop. Fortunately for them, the Connors and their colleagues left northern Mexico and took their high-fat diet with them. Once the scientists were gone, the Tarahumara went back to their old ways. High-fat foods were no longer available, which meant that, once again, the Tarahumara's environment supported only one type of diet.

In the modern industrialized world, things are not so easy. McDonald's, Burger King, Wendy's, and Kentucky Fried Chicken are not going anywhere, so we have to rely on our awareness of the fat instinct and the behaviors that overcome it. It's also helpful if we're around people who reinforce healthful behaviors. In other words, spend time with friends who support your healthy lifestyle.

I guess the moral of this story is that it's important to establish your priorities and then discern whether or not your environment—and your friends—are supporting your goals. It's important for you to have friends who, at the very least, understand what you are doing on the Pritikin Program, and support you while you are doing it. Ideally, you and your friends would all be on the program, but in this less-than-perfect world of ours, the best we can often hope for is understanding and respect. That's usually more than enough to maintain your healthy lifestyle and keep your friends.

STRATEGY #5: KNOW YOUR EMOTIONAL TRIGGERS

Finally, the day is done. You started out the day perhaps fourteen hours earlier with your oatmeal and a walk. Since then, a lot has happened. A seemingly endless series of demands have been placed upon you. You've been forced, either by your own internal needs or those of others, to be your best self, or your professional self, and now all you want to do is go home, put your feet up, and relax. Of course, relaxing for most of us means having something to eat.

I mentioned earlier that my discipline is strongest in the morning and weakest in the evening, which means that by the end of the day I'm most vulnerable to the fat instinct. This is the case even on my best days. But all of us have days that people older and wiser warned us about—days that threatened us, or made us feel badly about ourselves or what we do. Such situations elicit the fat instinct like the smell of raw meat awakens a lion.

The reason, simply, is that whenever we feel emotionally or psychologically threatened, the fat instinct is triggered. The fat instinct is an essential part of our will to survive. Evolution has taught us that we need calories in order to survive—and the more calories, the better. That lesson has been instilled into our genes. Anything we perceive to be a threat to our survival—from an argument with a spouse or loved one, to the possible loss of status, to conflicts on the job—triggers our will to survive, which in turn seems to bring the fat instinct out of its lair. Once the fat instinct is awakened, we're going to experience an increase in our desire for high-calorie foods and drinks. At the very least, we will be driven to overeat high-calorie foods, and at worst we will gorge.

In order to understand how to circumvent the fat instinct's influence on us, especially in emotionally threatening situations, we have to identify our high-risk situations, and our high-risk foods. High-risk foods are those rich in fat and processed calories that cause us to overeat or gorge. We have to know when we are vulnerable, and what we tend to eat in those situations.

At least 70 percent of the situations that cause us to overeat or choose foods on the basis of the fat instinct are known to us. In fact, they occur over and over again. One of the best things you can do for yourself is to take an inventory of all the places over the last month where you overindulged or flat out lost it. Examine the situation and reflect on why that situation makes you feel threatened or weak or hungry.

What most of us also know is that at the end of the day, when we are finally home and feeling safe, we eat, and usually keep on eating, until our fat instincts are fully sated.

Strategy #6: Make Your Home a Mini-Pritikin Center

My protection against losing it entirely at night is to have on hand lots of foods that satisfy me completely, but nothing that will trigger my fat instinct. There are lots of comfort foods that are fairly nnocuous, as well, such as soups, salsa and bean dip, which I have with baked corn chips; sorbet, instead of ice cream; chocolate without the fat; fruit and dried fruit. These foods satisfy me, but do not contain fat or cholesterol, and consequently dampen my fat instinct. I'm a lot less likely to overeat them, and even if I do, most of these foods are relatively low in calories. They're not going to put weight on me.

If I am going to splurge, I force myself to have to go outside my home to do it. That, of course, presents a certain amount of resistance against my getting up and going out, which cuts down on the number of times I actually do go out to satisfy my fat instinct. But even when I do go out, I try to moderate the extremes. I do that, of course, by choosing the food with the least amount of fat and sugar, and the most fiber and water. If I go off the program, I don't go all the way off.

I'm at my weakest at eight P.M. and therefore I know that whatever is in my house at nine will be in my stomach at ten. As my brother Kenny used to say: "If I went to bed at nine o'clock every night, I'd be twenty pounds lighter." Therefore, I try to have a wide array of healthy choices on hand. That way, I will be able to satisfy my hunger without engaging my fat instinct.

Of course, in order to have such foods in our house, my wife and I have to plan ahead and shop accordingly. We know in advance that we're going to be weak at night, and there's no point in fooling ourselves by thinking that that's going to change. I'm not going to have a sudden epiphany and become disciplined overnight. I'm forty-six years old and I've been on the Pritikin Program virtually all my life. I'm not perfect and that's unlikely to change any time soon. What I have to do is to have foods available in my house that are healthy and provide the fewest calories—foods that satisfy me—when I'm feeling weak.

I've also got my larger safety net, the primary strands of which are the five simple behaviors that form the foundation of the Pritikin Program. Exercise is one of the greatest antidotes to stress and feelings of depression and low self-esteem. I do it every day to keep my craving for carbohydrates, but also to work off stress and keep my mood elevated. It makes me feel good. I try to eat the right carbohydrates and limit my fat intake in order to maintain my health and weight. I eat frequently to keep hunger and the fat instinct at bay. That way, I'm not overwhelmed by cravings that would entice me to eat foods that throw me completely off the program. And I do all that I have said in this chapter as a way to maintain consistency. This is my net.

And the truth is that occasionally I still fall off the wagon. No program is foolproof. Yet, I can live comfortably with this approach for the rest of my life. I can find satiety and satisfaction on this program virtually any day of the week, and any time of the day. There's plenty of flexibility on the program; I don't have to live according to a rigid set of rules that would restrict my schedule or travel in any way. And all of it gives me the rewards I have described in this book.

No program is perfect, however, because none of us are perfect. Occasionally, all of us stray from our ideals. That's part of what makes us human and even interesting. As I have tried to stress, we are not concerned with perfection so much as consistency. If you follow our recommendations consistently, you will experience all the rewards of good health, abundant energy, optimal weight, and enhanced appearance. Good health flows from a lifestyle that supports your genetic makeup, a way of life that our ancestors regarded as the normal human pattern. Today we call it the Pritikin Program.

RECIPES

Salmon and Mushroom Risotto
Sea Bass with Asparagus Cream
  Sauce
Shiitake Mushroom Stroganoff
Soupe au Pistou
Stuffed Potatoes
Spinach Roll-Ups

Szechuan Tofu and Fried Rice
Tuna Salad
Turkey Breast Meat Loaf
Vegetable Couscous
Vegetarian Meat Loaf
White Beans and Tomato Soup with
  Parsley Pesto

APRICOT RICE PILAF

Juice of 1 large orange (about ¼ cup juice)
1 cup diced celery
1 cup chopped onion
Grated zest of 2 oranges
½ cup sliced water chestnuts
12 dried apricots, cut into slivers
¼ teaspoon (freshly ground) black pepper
1 tablespoon low-sodium soy sauce
1½ cups cooked brown rice
1½ cups cooked wild rice
2 to 3 tablespoons unseasoned rice vinegar

Pour the orange juice into a large skillet, add the celery and onion, and cook over medium heat for 2 minutes.

Add the orange peel, water chestnuts, dried apricots, pepper, and soy sauce and cook, stirring occasionally, until the vegetables are tender.

Add the cooked rices and stir until well combined and the rice is heated through. Sprinkle with the rice vinegar, mix well, and serve.

Serves 6

Per serving: 155 calories, 34.5 g carbohydrate, 4.2 g protein, less than 1 g total fat, 0 mg cholesterol, 124 mg sodium, 2.8 g dietary fiber, 4% calories from fat

BALSAMIC STRAWBERRIES AND APPLES

3 cups strawberries, hulled and halved
2 medium sweet apples, such as Fuji or Delicious,
    peeled and cut into 1/2-inch cubes
1/4 cup apple juice concentrate
3 tablespoons orange juice
2 tablespoons balsamic vinegar
Grated zest of 1 orange

Combine the strawberries and apples in a large nonaluminum (nonreactive) bowl.

In a small bowl, mix together the apple juice concentrate, orange juice, and balsamic vinegar. Pour the mixture over the fruit, add the orange peel, and mix well but gently.

Marinate the fruit for 15 to 30 minutes, turning the fruit in the marinade occasionally.

Serve chilled or at room temperature.

Serves 8

Per serving: 57 calories, 14 g carbohydrate, less than 1 g protein, less than 1 g total fat, 0 mg cholesterol, 2 mg sodium, 2 g dietary fiber, 5% calories from fat

BANANA–CARROT–OAT BRAN MUFFINS

1³/₄ cups oat bran
³/₄ cup whole wheat flour
1 tablespoon low-sodium baking powder
1 cup nonfat milk
1 medium ripe banana
³/₄ cup grated carrot
¹/₂ cup date sugar
3 tablespoons barley malt or molasses
¹/₂ cup raisins or currants
¹/₂ cup egg substitute

Preheat the oven to 350 degrees.

Spray a 12-muffin pan with food release.

Combine the oat bran, flour, and baking powder in a large mixing bowl and stir in the milk.

In a separate bowl, mash the banana. Mix in the carrot, sugar, barley malt, raisins, and egg substitute. Stir into the oat bran mixture just until combined. Don't overmix.

Spoon the mixture into the prepared muffin pan. Bake at 350 degrees for 25 to 30 minutes or until a toothpick inserted into the center comes out clean.

Makes 12 large muffins or 36 minimuffins

Per large muffin: 143 calories, 23 g carbohydrate, 5 g protein, 1 g total fat, less than 1 g saturated fat, less than 1 mg cholesterol, 37 mg sodium, 3 g dietary fiber, 10% calories from fat

BLACK BEAN STEW

1½ medium onions, chopped
2 garlic cloves, minced
⅓ cup low-sodium vegetable or chicken broth
1 large stalk celery, sliced
1 large green bell pepper, diced
1 jalapeño chili pepper, seeded and finely chopped
2 medium tomatoes, chopped
3 cans (15 ounces each) salt-free black beans (reserve liquid;
    see Note)
¾ cup red wine
½ teaspoon dried thyme
1 teaspoon dried oregano
2 tablespoons low-sodium soy sauce
2 tablespoons red wine vinegar

In a large heavy-bottom Dutch oven or soup pot, sauté the onions and garlic in the broth for 2 to 3 minutes. Add the celery, bell pepper, and jalapeño pepper and cook over medium heat, covered, for 5 or 6 minutes, stirring occasionally, then add the tomatoes and cook for 1 minute more.

Add the canned beans, including the liquid, red wine, herbs, soy sauce, and vinegar. Cover the pot and cook over medium-low heat, stirring occasionally, until the vegetables are tender and the flavors well blended. Add a little extra vegetable stock if it becomes too dry.

Serve hot in shallow bowls, garnished with a dollop of nonfat sour cream or yogurt if desired.

Makes 10 cups

Per 1 cup: 146 calories, 25 g carbohydrate, 8 g protein, less than 1 g total fat, 0 mg cholesterol, 140 mg sodium, 7 g dietary fiber, 4% calories from fat

Note: If you can't find salt-free canned beans, rinse regular canned beans and use low-sodium vegetable broth, instead of the liquid in the can. Eliminate the soy sauce in the recipe to compensate for the additional sodium in the beans. You can also substitute your own cooked dried beans and their cooking liquid.

BRAISED PORK TENDERLOIN MEDALLIONS WITH APPLES AND PRUNES

18 pitted prunes
1 cup dry red wine
$1/2$ teaspoon cornstarch
1 cup fat-free, low-sodium chicken broth
1 tablespoon low-sodium soy sauce
2 tablespoons balsamic vinegar
$1 1/2$ pounds pork tenderloin, trimmed of all fat and sliced into
   $1/2$-inch thick medallions
$1/2$ cup all-purpose white flour
3 medium garlic cloves, minced
$1/4$ teaspoon white pepper
2 tart apples, such as Granny Smith, peeled, cored, and thinly sliced
3 tablespoons evaporated milk (optional)

Simmer the prunes and red wine in a small covered saucepan for about 5 minutes, or until the prunes are softened. Set aside. Combine the cornstarch with 1 tablespoon of the broth, mix in the soy sauce and balsamic vinegar, and set the mixture aside.

Pat the pork medallions dry with paper towels and dredge them in the flour, shaking off the excess (don't do this until you are ready to cook them). Spray a 12-inch nonstick skillet with cooking spray, heat over medium-high heat, and brown the pork on both sides. While the pork is browning add the garlic to the pan and sprinkle with white pepper.

Remove the skillet from the heat for a few minutes to cool off the pan, lower the heat to medium, and put the skillet back on the heat. Pour the wine and prunes into the skillet and add $1/2$ cup of the remaining broth. Break up the prunes with a wooden spoon as they cook and then add the apple slices. Cook, stirring occasionally, for a few minutes until the apples become limp and the sauce starts to thicken; add more broth if it becomes too dry.

Stir the cornstarch mixture and add it to the skillet. Cook and stir for a few minutes until the sauce becomes thick and glossy. Add the evaporated milk, if desired, to give the sauce a creamy look. Serve hot with rice, pasta, or potatoes.

Serves 6

Per serving: 291 calories, 36 g carbohydrate, 5 g total fat, 1.6 g saturated fat, 60 mg cholesterol, 195 mg sodium, 3.6 g dietary fiber, 13% calories from fat

CHICKEN CURRY

1 pound skinless chicken breast, cut into 1½-inch chunks
   (3 to 4 half-breasts)
½ cup dry white wine
1 cup chopped onion
2 garlic cloves, minced
1 cup sliced celery
1 cup sliced mushrooms
1 large tart green apple, cored and diced
2 tablespoons cornstarch
1½ cups low-sodium, fat-free chicken broth
1 to 2 teaspoons mild curry powder
1 tablespoon white wine Worcestershire sauce
⅔ cup nonfat milk powder
½ cup frozen peas, defrosted

In a large skillet over medium heat, cook the chicken pieces in the wine until the chicken is just white (three to five minutes). Remove the chicken with a slotted spoon and set aside.

To the liquid remaining in the pan (add 1 or 2 tablespoons of wine, more if necessary), add the onion and garlic and cook for 2 minutes. Add the celery and mushrooms and cook, stirring occasionally, for 2 minutes more. Add the apple and cook for an additional minute or two.

Stir the cornstarch into the broth and make sure it dissolves completely. Stir in the curry powder, Worcestershire sauce, and the milk powder, and mix until any lumps have dissolved.

Add the broth mixture to the vegetables in the skillet a cup at a time, stirring until the mixture thickens a little. When all the mixture has been used, add the cooked chicken pieces and the peas. Cook and stir until the curry is thick and creamy and the chicken is heated through.

Serves 6

*Per serving: 189 calories, 17 g carbohydrate, 22 g protein, 2 g total
fat, less than 1 g saturated fat, 46 mg cholesterol, 169 mg sodium,
2.5 g dietary fiber, 9% calories from fat*

BULGUR PILAF

1 cup chopped onion (1 medium)
1 cup chopped celery
2 cups sliced mushrooms
1 garlic clove, minced
2¼ cups defatted, low-sodium chicken or vegetable broth
1 teaspoon poultry seasoning
½ teaspoon dried oregano
1 cup bulgur
1 tablespoon Worcestershire sauce
1 tablespoon low-sodium soy sauce
¼ cup diced red bell pepper or pimiento
2 tablespoons chopped parsley
1 to 2 tablespoons natural rice vinegar (optional)

In a medium nonstick skillet, sauté the onion, celery, mushrooms, and garlic in ¼ cup of the broth until the vegetables are somewhat tender (3 to 4 minutes).

Stir in the poultry seasoning, oregano, and bulgur and mix well. Combine the remaining 2 cups broth with the Worcestershire and soy sauces and add to the skillet. Mix well and cook, covered, over a low heat for about 25 minutes, or until all the liquid has been absorbed. Stir in the chopped red pepper or pimiento and parsley. Season the pilaf with a sprinkling of rice vinegar, if desired.

Serve hot, at room temperature, or cold as a salad.

Serves 6

Per serving: 118 calories, 23 g carbohydrate, 6.4 g protein, less than 1 g total fat, 0 mg cholesterol, 154 mg sodium, 5.6 g dietary fiber, 4% calories from fat

CREAMY FRUIT AND BARLEY

2 cups cooked barley
1 cup halved strawberries
1 cup blueberries
1 cup sliced bananas
2 tablespoons unsweetened fruit spread
1 cup nonfat plain yogurt

Combine the cooked barley and fruit.

Stir the fruit spread into the yogurt. Add the yogurt mixture to the barley and fruit and mix gently until well combined.

Serve at room temperature or cold.

Serves 8

Per serving: 98 calories, 22 g carbohydrates, 2.8 g protein, less than 1 g total fat, less than 1 mg cholesterol, 29 mg sodium, 2.7 g dietary fiber, 4% calories from fat

FIESTA CORN SALAD

1½ cups cooked kidney beans, or 1 can (15 ounces) low-sodium
   beans, rinsed and drained
1 package (10 ounces) frozen corn kernels, thawed
⅔ cup salsa, such as Enrico's salt-free
½ cup chopped green bell pepper

Combine all ingredients; mix well. Refrigerate up to 1 week.

Makes eight ½-cup servings

Per serving: 86 calories, 18 g carbohydrate, 4 g protein, less than 1 g total fat, 0 mg cholesterol, 54 mg sodium, 4 g dietary fiber, 2% calories from fat

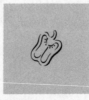

FISH FILLETS WITH ORANGE SALSA

½ cup unsweetened orange juice
2 to 3 tablespoons mild salsa, such as Enrico's salt-free
Mild Chunky Salsa
10 to 12 ounces fish fillets, such as orange roughy, sole, or halibut
½ cup all-purpose white flour
2 tablespoons chopped green onions

In a small bowl, combine the orange juice and salsa and set aside. Dry the fish fillets thoroughly with paper towels.

Spray an 11-inch nonstick skillet with nonstick cooking spray and put the pan over high heat. Dredge the fish fillets in the flour, shaking off the excess, and sauté on one side until they are lightly browned (2 to 3 minutes). Using 2 spatulas, gently turn the fillets over and brown for 2 minutes on the other side. Don't try to move the fillets around in the pan as they will probably stick. Remove the pan from the heat and allow it to cool off a little before continuing.

Stir up the salsa mixture and pour it over the fish (the fish will unstick easily). Lower the heat to medium and cook for 4 to 5 minutes, basting with the sauce once in a while, until the fish is cooked through and the sauce has been reduced to a thick glaze.

Garnish the fish with a sprinkling of green onions and serve.

Serves 2

Per serving: 243 calories, 33 g carbohydrate, 25 g protein, 10 g total fat, less than 1 g saturated fat, 28 mg cholesterol, 131 mg sodium, less than 1 g dietary fiber, 28% calories from fat

Fish Fillets with Citrus Sauce

1/4 cup natural rice vinegar
1/4 cup dry white wine
2 tablespoons frozen pineapple concentrate, defrosted
2 tablespoons unsweetened orange marmalade
1 tablespoon Dijon mustard (low-sodium if possible)
1 tablespoon white wine Worcestershire sauce
Peel of 1 lemon, cut into thin strips
Peel of 1/2 orange, cut into thin strips
1 tablespoon lemon juice
1 1/4 pounds fish fillets
1/2 cup all-purpose white flour
1 tablespoon chopped parsley

In a small nonreactive (not aluminum) saucepan, cook the vinegar until it is reduced by about half. Add the wine, pineapple concentrate, marmalade, mustard, Worcestershire sauce, lemon and orange peel, and lemon juice. Cook over medium heat for about 1 minute until the marmalade is dissolved and the sauce is slightly syrupy. Set aside.

Dry the fish fillets very well between pieces of paper towel. Spray a nonstick skillet with nonstick cooking spray, such as Pam and heat until hot.

Dredge the fillets with flour, shaking off the excess, and add them to the pan. Brown the fish on both sides. Remove the pan from the heat and allow it to cool off a little before continuing.

Return the pan to the heat and pour the sauce over the browned fillets. Simmer over medium-low heat, basting the fish occasionally, until the fish is cooked through (about 3 to 4 minutes), and the sauce has thickened.

Sprinkle with chopped parsley and serve.

Serves 4

Per serving: 218 calories, 18 g carbohydrate, 18 g protein, 8 g total fat, less than 1 g saturated fat, 22 mg cholesterol, 111 mg sodium, 1 g dietary fiber, 33% calories from fat

FISH FILLETS WITH RED ONION, TOMATOES, AND CAPERS

¼ cup dry white wine
Juice of 2 limes (about ¼ cup)
2 garlic cloves, chopped or put through a garlic press
1 large red onion, coarsely chopped
2 large tomatoes, seeded and diced
1 jalapeño chili pepper, seeded and finely chopped
3 tablespoons well-rinsed capers
1¼ pounds fish fillets, such as orange roughy, sea bass, or halibut

Pour the white wine and lime juice into a large skillet. Add the garlic and red onion and cook, covered, over medium heat for 3 minutes.

Add the tomatoes, jalapeño, and capers, mix well, and cook, covered, for 1 minute.

Add the fish fillets to the pan and cover them with the vegetables. Cook, covered, over medium-low heat, basting occasionally with pan juices, until the fish is cooked through (5 to 8 minutes, depending on the thickness of the fish). The fish is done when it flakes easily with a fork.

Lift the fillets gently out of the pan with a spatula and serve each one strewn with some of the vegetables from the pan.

The fish may be garnished with a sprinkling of fresh chopped parsley or cilantro if desired.

Serves 4

Per serving: 201 calories, 11 g carbohydrate, 18 g protein, 8 g total fat, less than 1 g saturated fat, 22 mg cholesterol, 233 mg sodium, 2 g dietary fiber, 37% calories from fat

GINGER MARMALADE CHICKEN

6 skinless chicken breast halves, all fat removed
$1/2$ cup sugar-free orange marmalade
2 teaspoons Dijon mustard (low-sodium if possible)
1 tablespoon white wine Worcestershire sauce
1 tablespoon low-sodium soy sauce
2 tablespoons natural rice vinegar
1 tablespoon chopped fresh gingerroot
1 teaspoon cornstarch dissolved in 1 tablespoon cold water

Preheat the oven to 400 degrees.

Place the chicken breasts side by side in a shallow baking dish just large enough to hold them without overlapping. Combine the marmalade, mustard, Worcestershire sauce, soy sauce, vinegar, and ginger until well mixed and spoon it evenly over the chicken breasts.

Bake uncovered at 400 degrees for 20 to 25 minutes, or until the chicken is cooked through and golden brown on top.

Carefully pour the liquid from the baking dish into a small saucepan set over medium heat. Stir up the cornstarch mixture and add it to the saucepan. Cook and stir until the marmalade sauce has thickened.

Serve each chicken breast napped with hot marmalade sauce.

Serves 6

Per serving: 199 calories, 19 g carbohydrate, 26.6 g protein, 1.5 g total fat, less than 1/2 g saturated fat, 65.8 mg cholesterol, 202 mg sodium, 1.3 g dietary fiber, 7% calories from fat

GINGERED WINTER SQUASH SOUP

1/4 cup dry white wine
1 cup medium chopped onion
1 tablespoon fresh chopped gingerroot
1/2 teaspoon ground cumin
1/2 teaspoon dry mustard powder
1/4 teaspoon ground mace
1/4 teaspoon ground cinnamon
1/4 teaspoon black pepper
3 cups cubed peeled butternut squash (about 1 1/2 pounds)
1 cup cubed peeled sweet potato (about 1/2 medium)
3/4 cup sliced parsnip (about 1 1/2 parsnips)
3 cans (15 ounces each) low-sodium chicken stock
1 tablespoon Worcestershire sauce
1 tablespoon low-sodium soy sauce
1 1/2 tablespoons natural rice vinegar
2 tablespoons chopped parsley or snipped chives
    (for garnish)

Put the wine into a large (6-quart) saucepan or Dutch oven over medium heat. Add the onion, ginger, cumin, mustard powder, mace, cinnamon, and black pepper, and sauté for several minutes, or until the onion is somewhat tender.

Add the squash, sweet potato, parsnip, and stock. Bring to a boil, reduce the heat, and simmer, partially covered, about 30 minutes or until the vegetables are tender.

Puree the soup (in 2 batches) in a processor and pour the puree into a 3-quart saucepan.

Stir in the Worcestershire sauce, soy sauce, and rice vinegar. Reheat the mixture, stirring constantly, and serve hot.

Garnish with a sprinkling of parsley or chives.

Makes six 1-cup servings

Per serving: 120 calories, 20 g carbohydrate, 6 g protein, 1.5 g total fat, less than 1 g saturated fat, 0 mg cholesterol, 140 mg sodium, 1.6 g dietary fiber, 11% calories from fat

Golden Pea and Sweet Potato Soup

1/4 cup dry white wine
1 onion, chopped
1 jalapeño chili pepper, seeded and minced
1 tablespoon minced fresh gingerroot
2 teaspoons ground cumin
2 teaspoons ground coriander
1/2 teaspoon ground turmeric
1/2 teaspoon ground cinnamon
7 cups (or more) defatted low-sodium chicken or
   vegetable broth
1 large sweet potato, peeled and diced
1 cup dried yellow split peas

Pour the wine into a large heavy saucepan or Dutch oven. Add the onion and jalapeño and cook, covered, over medium heat until tender, 3 to 4 minutes. Stir in the ginger, cumin, coriander, turmeric, and cinnamon and cook for 1 minute.

Add the broth, sweet potato, and peas. Bring the mixture to a boil, reduce the heat to medium-low, cover, and simmer until the sweet potato and peas are very tender (about 1 to 1 1/2 hours), stirring once in a while.

Pour the contents of the saucepan into a processor and process until smooth (you may have to do this in 2 batches to prevent leakage from the processor).

Return the pureed soup to the saucepan, reheat, and serve. Thin the soup with extra broth if necessary.

To serve, top with 1 tablespoon of nonfat yogurt and a sprinkling of chopped cilantro; or serve in shallow soup bowls, sprinkled with chopped chives or parsley; or garnish with a swirl of red pepper puree.

Makes eight 1-cup servings

*Per serving: 142 calories, 14 g carbohydrate, 5 g protein, 2 g total fat,
less than 1 g saturated fat, 0 mg cholesterol, 51 mg sodium, 5 g
dietary fiber, 17% calories from fat*

Note: This soup is very low in sodium and would be a good choice
for people with hypertension.

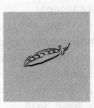

GOLDEN RICE

¼ cup unsweetened pineapple juice
1 tablespoon low-sodium soy sauce
1 tablespoon Worcestershire sauce
½ teaspoon turmeric powder
1½ teaspoons apple juice concentrate
1 tablespoon rice vinegar
½ medium onion, finely chopped
1 tablespoon chopped or grated gingerroot
2 garlic cloves, crushed or minced
¼ cup low-sodium vegetable or chicken broth
4 cups cooked brown rice
½ cup frozen or fresh peas
½ cup diced red bell pepper

In a small bowl, mix together the pineapple juice, soy sauce, Worcestershire sauce, turmeric, apple juice concentrate, and vinegar until the turmeric is completely dissolved. Set aside.

In a large nonstick skillet, sauté the onion, ginger, and garlic in the broth until the onion is tender. Stir in the cooked rice and mix well.

Add the pineapple-turmeric mixture and cook over low heat, stirring, until the rice has taken on a creamy, yellow color. Add a little extra stock if it gets too dry.

Stir in the peas and the red pepper. Mix well and cook until the rice and peas are heated through.

Serve hot as a side dish or cold as a rice salad (you may wish to sprinkle on extra vinegar if it is used as a salad).

Serves 8

Per serving: 136 calories, 28 g carbohydrate, 3.8 g protein, 1 g total fat, 0 g saturated fat, 0 mg cholesterol, 108 mg sodium, 3 g dietary fiber, 7% calories from fat

PIÑA COLADA ICE CREAM

2 large ripe but firm bananas, peeled
1 can (20 ounces) pineapple chunks packed in juice, drained
1 teaspoon coconut extract
¼ cup nonfat milk

Put the bananas into a plastic bag and freeze them. Spread the pineapple chunks on a cookie sheet lined with cooking parchment paper and freeze.

When the bananas are frozen, cut them into chunks with a sharp knife. Put the frozen banana slices and frozen pineapple into a food processor fitted with the steel chopping blade. Add the coconut extract and milk. Process until smooth.

Serve immediately.

Serves 8

Per serving: 62 calories, 16 g carbohydrate, less than 1 g protein, less than 1 g total fat, less than 1 mg cholesterol, 6 mg sodium, 2 g dietary fiber, 3% calories from fat

Note: To refreeze, put the ice cream into a plastic container. Cover with plastic wrap and press the wrap down so that it touches the ice cream. The idea is to prevent air from getting to the ice cream and causing it to frost over.

Place the lid on the container and freeze. You will have to allow the ice cream to soften again before you serve it, or put it back into the processor to soften it more quickly.

HARVEST VEGETABLE STEW

2 large garlic cloves
1 medium onion, diced
1 teaspoon dried thyme
1/4 cup defatted low-sodium chicken or vegetable broth
1 medium yam or sweet potato, peeled and cut into
    1-inch pieces
4 medium red potatoes, scrubbed and cut into 1-inch pieces
1 medium (about 1 pound) butternut squash, peeled, seeded,
    and cut into 1-inch pieces
1 can (12 ounces) low-sodium V8
1/2 cup red wine
2 bay leaves
1 tablespoon low-sodium soy sauce
1/4 teaspoon red pepper flakes
1/2 cup water (optional)
2 cups cauliflowerettes
1 can (8 ounces) salt-free kidney beans, drained
4 green onions, chopped

In a 6-quart stew pot or Dutch oven, simmer the garlic, onion, and thyme together in the broth until the mixture is fragrant (about 3 minutes).

Add the yam, red potatoes, squash, V8, red wine, bay leaves, soy sauce, and pepper flakes. Bring to a boil, cover the pot, and reduce the heat. Simmer over medium-low heat for about 20 minutes. Check the liquid; if it is beginning to look too dry, add the water.

Add the cauliflower and cook for 10 minutes more. Add the kidney beans and cook until the beans are heated through and the rest of the vegetables are tender.

Sprinkle with green onions and serve hot.

Serves 6

Per serving: 245 calories, 52 g carbohydrate, 7 g protein, less than 1 g total fat, 0 mg cholesterol, 138 mg sodium, 7 g dietary fiber, 2% calories from fat

POTATOES WITH FENNEL AND TOMATOES

1 large onion, chopped
1 large fennel bulb (about 1 pound), sliced white part only
1 large garlic clove, minced
¼ cup dry white wine or low-sodium vegetable stock
1 pound red potatoes, scrubbed and sliced (about 6 small)
6 medium tomatoes, seeded and diced
1 bay leaf
⅛ teaspoon saffron or turmeric powder
1 teaspoon dried thyme
½ cup low-sodium V8 juice
½ cup water or white wine
Freshly ground black pepper

In a large skillet over medium heat, cook the onion, fennel, and garlic in the wine until the onion is soft (approximately five minutes).

Add the potatoes, tomatoes, bay leaf, saffron, and thyme and mix thoroughly. Stir in the V8 and water. Turn the heat to medium-low and cook, covered, stirring occasionally, for about 30 minutes, or until the vegetables are soft.

Season with black pepper and serve hot or at room temperature.

Serves 6

Per serving: 129 calories, 25 g carbohydrate, 3.6 g protein, less than 1 g total fat, 0 mg cholesterol, 39 mg sodium, 3.5 g dietary fiber, 4% calories from fat

PUMPKIN CUSTARD

1 can (16 ounces) pumpkin
1/2 cup date sugar
1 1/4 cups evaporated skim milk
1/4 cup apple juice concentrate
1/2 teaspoon pumpkin pie spice
1/4 teaspoon cinnamon
1/2 cup egg whites (4 egg whites)

Combine all ingredients in a food processor or blender, or use an electric mixer.

Spray a 9-inch pie dish with food release, pour in the pumpkin puree, and level it off with a spatula.

Bake at 375 degrees for approximately 40 minutes, or until the custard is set.

Allow to cool and then refrigerate.

Serves 6

Per serving: 139 calories, 26 g carbohydrate, 7 g protein, 1 g total fat, less than 1 g saturated fat, 2 mg cholesterol, 108 mg sodium, 2 g dietary fiber, 6% calories from fat

Note: To prevent the pumpkin custard or pie from splitting as it cools, turn off the oven and allow the pie to cool in the oven for at least 30 minutes with the *oven door open.*

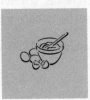

RED PEPPER—LENTIL STEW

1/2 cup dried lentils
1 large onion, chopped
1/4 cup water or low-sodium vegetable stock
3 large red bell peppers, seeded and diced
1 teaspoon dried basil
1 teaspoon dried marjoram
1/2 teaspoon dried thyme
1/4 to 1/2 teaspoon cayenne pepper
1/8 teaspoon white pepper
2 cups low-sodium vegetable broth
1/4 cup dry red wine
1/4 cup dry sherry
1 cup cooked white beans, or 1 can (8 ounces) low-sodium beans, drained
2 tablespoons tomato paste
1/4 cup chopped fresh parsley

Rinse and drain the lentils and set aside.

In a large deep saucepan (about 3 quarts), sauté the onion over medium heat in the water until softened somewhat. Add the bell peppers, basil, marjoram, thyme, cayenne, and white pepper. Cook for 2 minutes longer, or until the flavors are well blended, adding a tablespoon or two of water if it starts to look too dry.

Pour in the broth, red wine, sherry, and lentils. Bring to a boil, lower the heat, and simmer gently, covered, for 30 to 40 minutes, or until the lentils are soft and the liquid has thickened.

Add the cooked or canned beans, stir in the tomato paste, and cook several minutes longer, until the tomato paste is well blended.

Stir in the chopped parsley and serve either hot or at room temperature.

Serves 4

Per serving: 200 calories, 36 g carbohydrate, 16 g protein, less than 1 g total fat, less than 1 g saturated fat, 0 mg cholesterol, 26 mg sodium, 13 g dietary fiber, 3% calories from fat

SALMON PÂTÉ

1/2 cup rinsed fat-free cottage cheese or fat-free ricotta
1 can (15 ounces) red salmon, salt-free or well rinsed, skin removed
3 water-packed artichoke hearts, rinsed and drained
2 scallions
6 drops Tabasco
1 teaspoon Dijon mustard, salt-free
1 tablespoon lemon juice
2 ounces pimiento, drained
2 to 3 tablespoons fresh chopped dill, or 1 tablespoon dried
1 tablespoon well-rinsed capers

Blend the cottage cheese in a food processor until it is smooth.

Add the salmon, artichoke hearts, scallions, Tabasco, mustard, and lemon juice and process, using short pulses, until everything is combined and coarsely chopped.

Add the pimiento, dill, and capers and using short pulses, process again, so that there are still some pieces of pimiento showing.

Chill or serve at room temperature as an hors d'oeuvre spread for crackers or raw vegetables. It also makes a great sandwich spread.

Makes 2 1/2 cups (ten 1/4-cup servings)

Per serving: 86 calories, 2 g carbohydrate, 9 g protein, 4 g total fat, 1 g saturated fat, 11 mg cholesterol, 113 mg sodium, 1 g dietary fiber, 45% calories from fat

SHRIMP AND PINEAPPLE RICE

1 can (20 ounces) unsweetened pineapple chunks, packed in juice
1 tablespoon low-sodium soy sauce
$1/2$ teaspoon turmeric powder
$1 1/2$ teaspoons apple juice concentrate
$1/2$ pound raw medium shrimp, shelled and cleaned (or use frozen)
2 medium garlic cloves, minced
4 cups cooked brown rice
3 green onions, sliced
1 medium jalapeño chili pepper, seeded and finely chopped
$1/2$ cup thin-sliced red bell pepper

Drain the pineapple chunks, reserving the juice, and set aside. In a small bowl combine the soy sauce, turmeric, apple juice concentrate, and 1 tablespoon of the reserved pineapple juice. Set aside.

In a large skillet, cook the shrimp with the garlic in $1/3$ cup of the reserved pineapple juice until the shrimp are just opaque (2 to 3 minutes). Remove the shrimp with a slotted spoon and set aside.

To the liquid remaining in the pan add the cooked rice and stir-fry for 1 minute. Stir in the soy sauce–turmeric mixture and cook until the rice is yellow. Stir in the pineapple chunks, green onions, jalapeño, and red pepper and cook for about 1 minute. Add the shrimp and any collected juices to the pan, mix well, and cook until the shrimp are heated through.

Serve hot.

Serves 8

Per serving: 179 calories, 35 g carbohydrate, 7.5 g protein, 1.2 g total fat, negligible saturated fat, 41.5 mg cholesterol, 144 mg sodium, 2.5 g dietary fiber, 6% calories from fat

Spicy Raspberry Chicken

---

6 to 12 small chicken breast halves, trimmed of all fat
4 ounces sugar-free raspberry preserves
3 ounces frozen pineapple juice concentrate, defrosted
1 tablespoon low-sodium soy sauce
1 tablespoon rice vinegar
2 tablespoons lemon juice
2 garlic cloves, minced
1 tablespoon minced fresh gingerroot, or 1$\frac{1}{2}$ teaspoons
   ginger power
$\frac{1}{2}$ teaspoon dried basil
$\frac{1}{8}$ teaspoon chili powder
$\frac{1}{8}$ teaspoon curry powder
$\frac{1}{4}$ to $\frac{1}{2}$ teaspoon crushed, dried hot red pepper flakes
Dash of Tabasco
1 teaspoon cornstarch dissolved in 1 tablespoon cold water

Preheat oven to 400 degrees.

Place the chicken breasts side by side in a shallow baking dish just
large enough to hold them without overlapping. Combine all the
remaining ingredients and spoon over the chicken breasts. There is
enough sauce for 12 chicken breasts, so if you use only 6, use half the
sauce and refrigerate or freeze the remainder.

Bake the chicken, uncovered, at 400 degrees for 20 to 30 minutes,
depending on the thickness of the breasts.

When the chicken is done, carefully pour off the sauce from the
baking dish into a small saucepan and place it over medium heat. Stir
up the cornstarch and water mixture and add it to the sauce. Cook,
stirring constantly, until the sauce has slightly thickened and turned
shiny (2 to 3 minutes).

Serve each chicken breast hot, napped with a little of the sauce,
accompanied with rice or potatoes and a green vegetable.

Serves 6 to 12

Per serving: 173 calories, 8 g carbohydrate, 27 g protein, 3 g total fat, less than 1 g saturated fat, 72 mg cholesterol, 125 mg sodium, less than 1 g dietary fiber, 17% calories from fat

Summer Chicken Salad

6 tablespoons lime juice (from 3 limes)
2 tablespoons barley malt
1 tablespoon low-sodium soy sauce
$1/8$ to $1/4$ teaspoon crushed, dried hot red pepper flakes
2 teaspoons minced gingerroot
3 poached chicken breasts, skinned and cut into 1-inch pieces
$1/2$ large cucumber, peeled, seeded, and cut into $1/2$-inch cubes
1 red bell pepper, cut into $1/2$-inch pieces
1 papaya, peeled, seeded, and cut into $1/2$-inch cubes
1 cup dried dates, sliced lengthwise
2 green onions, sliced, including green tops
$1/4$ cup chopped fresh mint

In a medium bowl, combine the lime juice, barley malt, soy sauce, red pepper flakes, and ginger until the barley malt has completely dissolved. Add the chicken pieces and toss to coat the chicken thoroughly with the marinade (you can do this several hours ahead of time).

In a large bowl, gently mix together the cucumber, red bell pepper, papaya, dates, and green onions.

Add the marinated chicken plus any excess marinade and the chopped mint. Toss carefully until the ingredients are well combined.

Chill or serve at room temperature.

Serves 6

Per serving: 206 calories, 40 g carbohydrate, 11 g protein, less than 1 g total fat, 24 mg cholesterol, 135 mg sodium, 4 g dietary fiber, 4% calories from fat

Note: Cantaloupe, pineapple chunks, orange slices, peaches, or nectarines can be substituted for the papaya. The salad can be served in a bowl lined with red leaf lettuce or piled into a scooped-out cantaloupe, papaya, or pineapple half.

SWEET POTATO SPICE MUFFINS

2 cups whole wheat pastry or cake flour
1 teaspoon baking soda
1 tablespoon low-sodium baking powder (Featherweight)
1/2 teaspoon ginger powder
1 teaspoon allspice
1 teaspoon cinnamon
1/2 cup date sugar
4 egg whites
2 jars (6 ounces each) pureed sweet potato, or use baby food
1/4 cup mild-flavored molasses
3/4 cup 1% buttermilk
1/2 cup raisins

Preheat the oven to 375 degrees. Spray a muffin tin with nonstick cooking spray.

In a large bowl, mix together the flour, baking soda, baking powder, spices, and date sugar.

In a medium bowl, beat the egg whites until slightly frothy. Stir in the sweet potato puree, molasses, and buttermilk.

Stir the sweet potato mixture into the flour mixture and fold in the raisins. Do not overmix.

Spoon the batter evenly into the prepared muffin tin. Bake at 375 degrees for 25 to 30 minutes, or until a toothpick inserted in the center comes out clean.

Makes 12 large muffins or 36 minimuffins

Per large muffin: 154 calories, 34 g carbohydrate, 5 g protein, less than 1 g total fat, less than 1 mg cholesterol, 152 mg sodium, 3 g dietary fiber, 6% calories from fat

SWEET AND SOUR CHICKEN

1 tablespoon chopped fresh ginger
2 minced garlic cloves
1 cup chopped onion
1 cup defatted low-sodium chicken broth
1/4 cup white wine
6 ounces unsweetened pineapple juice (use juice drained from
  pineapple chunks)
3 boneless, skinless chicken breast halves, cubed
1 tablespoon low-sodium soy sauce
1/4 teaspoon poultry seasoning
1 red bell pepper, thinly sliced
1 green bell pepper, thinly sliced
1 cup pineapple chunks, drained
1/4 cup tomato puree
1 tablespoon cornstarch
2 tablespoons water
1 tablespoon apple juice concentrate
1 tablespoon white wine Worcestershire sauce
1 tablespoon rice vinegar

In a medium skillet, simmer the ginger, garlic, onion, broth, and white wine, uncovered, for 10 minutes. Add the pineapple juice and simmer for 1 or 2 minutes more.

Add the chicken, soy sauce, seasoning, red and green peppers, pineapple chunks, and tomato puree. Simmer for 10 minutes, partially covered, stirring occasionally.

Dissolve the cornstarch in the water. Add the apple juice concentrate, Worcestershire sauce, and vinegar and mix well. Blend into the chicken mixture and simmer, stirring, until the sauce has thickened and becomes clear.

Serve hot over brown rice.

Serves 6

Per serving: 141 calories, 15 g protein, 1 g total fat, less than 1 g saturated fat, 33 mg cholesterol, 170 mg sodium, 2 g dietary fiber, 6% calories from fat

VEGETARIAN CHILI

1 medium red onion, chopped
2 garlic cloves, minced
1 stalk celery, sliced
1 medium carrot, diced
1 1/2 cups low-sodium vegetable broth, or defatted chicken broth
1 cup quartered mushrooms
1/2 cup frozen corn kernels
1/2 cup frozen lima beans
2 mild green canned chilies, seeded, rinsed, and finely chopped
2 1/2 teaspoons dried oregano
1 tablespoon chili powder
2 1/2 teaspoons cumin powder
2 large tomatoes, chopped
1 can (16 ounces) salt-free tomato sauce
3 cups cooked beans, or 2 cans (15 ounces each) salt-free
1 tablespoon low-sodium barbecue sauce
1 tablespoon Worcestershire sauce

In a large saucepan, cook the onion, garlic, celery, and carrot in 1/2 cup of the broth over medium heat for 5 minutes. Add the mushrooms, corn, lima beans, chilies, and seasonings. Cover and simmer over medium-low heat for 15 minutes.

Stir in the remaining 1 cup broth, tomatoes, tomato sauce, beans, barbecue sauce, and Worcestershire sauce. Cover and simmer for 15 to 20 minutes, stirring occasionally, adding a little additional vegetable broth if it gets too dry.

Serves 10

Per serving: 122 calories, 22 g carbohydrate, 7 g protein, less than 1 g fat, 0 mg cholesterol, 53 mg sodium, 6 g dietary fiber, 6% calories from fat

WHITE BEAN SPREAD OR DIP

1 can (15 ounces) salt-free white beans, drained
2 to 3 tablespoons lemon juice
2 to 4 garlic cloves, finely chopped or put through a garlic press
4 teaspoons white wine Worcestershire sauce (Lea & Perrins)
1 teaspoon Dijon mustard with horseradish
1 teaspoon rice vinegar
2 tablespoons chopped fresh parsley

Combine all ingredients except the parsley in a food processor or blender until smooth. Transfer the mixture into a bowl and stir in the hopped parsley.

Serve as a spread or dip, chilled or at room temperature, with rackers or raw vegetables.

Makes 1¹/₂ cups (six ¹/₄-cup servings)

Per ¹/₄-cup serving: 107 calories, 19 g carbohydrate, 7 g protein, less than 1 g total fat, less than 1 mg cholesterol, 43 mg sodium, 4 g dietary fiber, 3% calories from fat

WHITE BEANS WITH TOMATOES AND BASIL

1 medium red onion, finely diced
2 large garlic cloves, crushed or chopped
1/4 cup defatted chicken broth or white wine
1 medium red bell pepper, finely diced
2 medium tomatoes, seeded and finely diced
2 cans (15 ounces each) salt-free white beans, drained, or 3 cups
    cooked beans
3 tablespoons balsamic vinegar
1 tablespoon white wine Worcestershire sauce
1 tablespoon low-sodium soy sauce
1/4 teaspoon black pepper
3 tablespoons chopped fresh basil

In a medium skillet, cook the onion and garlic in the broth over medium heat for about 3 minutes, stirring. Add the chopped red pepper and cook for 2 minutes more. Add the tomatoes and beans, mix well, and cook, stirring occasionally, until heated through.

Combine the vinegar, Worcestershire sauce, and soy sauce and stir it into the bean mixture. Sprinkle in the black pepper, turn the heat to medium-low, and simmer, covered, for about 3 minutes, stirring occasionally. Mix in the chopped basil, and cook for a minute or two longer.

Serve hot or transfer the mixture to a bowl and allow to cool to room temperature (the flavors will be enhanced as it cools).

Serve as a side dish or a vegetarian entrée, or chilled as a salad.

Makes ten 1/2-cup servings

Per serving: 100 calories, 18 g carbohydrate, 6 g protein, less than 1 g total fat, 0 mg cholesterol, 82 mg sodium, 4 g dietary fiber, 3% calories from fat

BAKED YAMS

1 large yam or sweet potato
4 sheets of aluminum foil

Preheat the over to 400 degrees. Wash and scrub the yam, pat dry, and cut into 4 equal pieces. Wrap each piece of yam in a sheet of aluminum foil. Place the yams on a baking dish and bake for 30 to 40 minutes, or until yams are soft.

Serves 4

Per serving: 40 calories, 9 g carbohydrate, 0.5 g protein, less than 1 g total fat, 0 mg cholesterol, 3 mg sodium, 1.3 g dietary fiber

BEAN TOSTADAS

6 corn tortillas
1½ cups cooked pinto beans
1 garlic clove
½ cup minced red onion
1 teaspoon cumin powder
½ cup salt-free mild or hot salsa
1 tablespoon chopped cilantro
2 cups shredded lettuce
2 cups diced tomatoes
½ cup nonfat sour cream (optional)

Place the corn tortillas on a cookie sheet and bake at 400 degrees for 7 minutes, or until crisp. Set aside.

Place the pinto beans, garlic, red onion, cumin powder, salsa, and cilantro in a food processor. Blend until smooth.

Spread the bean mixture on the tortillas and top with the shredded lettuce and diced tomatoes. If desired, top with nonfat sour cream.

Serves 6

Per serving: 293 calories, 56 g carbohydrate, 15 g protein, 1.8 g total fat, 0.3 g saturated fat, 0 mg cholesterol, 72 mg sodium, 3.3 g dietary fiber, 5% calories from fat

BRAISED BRUSSELS SPROUTS

4 cups brussels sprouts
½ cup diced shallots
½ teaspoon minced garlic
1 teaspoon date sugar
½ tablespoon balsamic vinegar
Pinch of black pepper
Pinch of nutmeg
2 teaspoons lite soy sauce
1 tablespoon minced fresh parsley
½ cup vegetable broth

Steam the brussels sprouts for 10 minutes in boiling water. Set aside. Spray a little olive oil or Pam in a large nonstick pan and heat on medium heat. Sauté the shallots and garlic for 2 minutes.

Add the steamed brussels sprouts and date sugar and cook for 5 minutes, covered, on high heat. Add the balsamic vinegar, black pepper, nutmeg, and soy sauce. Cook for 5 minutes, uncovered, stirring frequently. Add the parsley and broth. Cook for 5 minutes more, uncovered.

Serves 4

Per serving: 112 calories, 22 g carbohydrate, 8 g protein, less than 1 g total fat, 0 mg cholesterol, 170 mg sodium, 8.6 g dietary fiber, 4% of calories from fat

BELGIAN CHICKEN STEW

---

1 cup diced carrots
2 cups sliced new potatoes
1/2 teaspoon minced garlic
1 cup diced brown onion
1 cup diced red bell pepper
2 cups diced mushrooms
1 bay leaf
2 cloves
Pinch of thyme
12 ounces chicken breasts, cut into 1-inch strips
1 cup dark beer
1 tablespoon tomato paste
1 1/2 tablespoons fruit spread
1 teaspoon red wine vinegar
1 tablespoon Dijon mustard
1 cup chicken broth
Pinch of black pepper
1 teaspoon chopped fresh tarragon
1 teaspoon cornstarch dissolved in 1 tablespoon cold water
   (optional)
2 tablespoons chopped parsley (for garnish)

In a 6-quart stew pot set over medium heat, steam the carrots and potatoes for 5 minutes in boiling water until crisp-tender. Set aside.

In a large skillet, sauté the garlic, onion, red pepper, mushrooms, bay leaf, cloves, thyme, and chicken in the beer for 10 minutes.

In a small bowl, mix the tomato paste, fruit spread, vinegar, mustard, and chicken broth. Stir into the chicken mixture.

Add the black pepper, tarragon, potatoes, and carrots and simmer, covered, for 10 minutes. Thicken with the cornstarch mixture, if necessary, and garnish with freshly chopped parsley.

Serves 4

Per serving: 353 calories, 32.4 g carbohydrate, 47.16 g protein, 2.93 g total fat, less than 1 g saturated fat, 102.8 mg cholesterol, 212 mg sodium, 4 g dietary fiber, 8% calories from fat

CHICKEN AND VEGETABLE SOUP

6 cups chicken broth
6 chicken breasts, diced, skinned, and boned
1 tablespoon minced garlic
1 cup diced carrots
1 cup diced celery
3/4 cup diced onion
1 cup diced leeks
2 cups diced tomatoes
2 teaspoons low-sodium soy sauce
Freshly ground black pepper to taste
1 teaspoon rice vinegar
Pinch of thyme
1 bay leaf
1 tablespoon chopped fresh parsley
1 tablespoon cornstarch diluted in 1 tablespoon cold water
1 recipe Matzo Balls (recipe follows)

Bring all ingredients, except diluted cornstarch and matzo balls, to a boil and simmer for 45 minutes.

Thicken with the cornstarch mixture. Add the matzo balls and keep warm.

Serves 10

MATZO BALLS

1/4 cup egg whites
1/4 cup chicken broth
1/3 cup matzo meal
2 cups chicken broth
1/2 teaspoon onion powder
1/4 cup chopped parsley
1 teaspoon low-sodium soy sauce

Beat the egg whites until foamy.

Mix the chicken broth, matzo meal, onion powder, parsley, and soy sauce. Add the egg whites and combine. Cover and chill for 2 hours or more.

Form into small balls (dip your hands in cold water to facilitate rolling).

In a 3-quart saucepan, bring chicken broth to a boil.

Drop the matzo balls one by one into boiling chicken broth, cover, and cook over low heat for 20 minutes.

Makes 12 matzo balls

Per serving: 103 calories, 9 g carbohydrate, 14 g protein, 0.76 g fat, 0.17 g saturated fat, 24 mg cholesterol, 151 mg sodium, 1.47 g dietary fiber, 6% calories from fat

CAESAR DRESSING

1 package Mori-Nu Lite tofu (ten ounces)
1 tablespoon Dijon mustard
1 teaspoon garlic powder
2/3 cup water
1 8-ounce bottle Pritikin Italian dressing
1 tablespoon balsamic vinegar
1 teaspoon rice vinegar
1 teaspoon lemon juice
1/2 teaspoon black pepper
1/2 teaspoon apple juice concentrate
1 teaspoon Worcestershire sauce
4 anchovies, rinsed

In an electric blender, blend all ingredients thoroughly. Refrigerate immediately.

Serves 16

Per 2-tablespoon serving: 14 calories, 1.48 g carbohydrate, 1.16 g protein, less than 1 g total fat, 0 mg cholesterol, 90 mg sodium, 0 g dietary fiber, 23% of calories from fat

CHICKEN FAJITAS

4 boneless, skinless chicken breasts (about 20 ounces)
1 1/2 tablespoons low-sodium soy sauce
1 tablespoon balsamic vinegar
1 teaspoon minced garlic
2 teaspoons minced jalapeño chili peppers
1/4 cup dry white wine
1 red onion, sliced
1 red bell pepper, cut into thin strips
1 green bell pepper, cut into thin strips
1 1/2 cups chopped tomatoes
1 tablespoon minced fresh cilantro or Italian parsley
1 tablespoon lime juice
6 corn tortillas

Cut the chicken breasts in 1/2-inch strips. Mix together the soy sauce and vinegar and marinate the chicken strips for a few minutes.

Spray a little olive oil or Pam on a large nonstick skillet and heat for 1 minute on medium heat. Sauté the garlic and jalapeños for 1 minute. Add the chicken strips and the marinade and cook, uncovered, over medium heat for 4 minutes, stirring occasionally (do not over-cook). Remove the chicken strips and set aside.

Add half of the white wine and sauté the onion and red and green peppers over medium heat for 3 minutes, adding the remaining wine if necessary. Add the tomatoes and cilantro and cook for 1 minute on high heat. Put the chicken back into the skillet and cook for 1 more minute on high heat, stirring frequently.

Just before serving, add the lime juice and serve with corn tortillas.

Serves 6

Per serving: 213 calories, 21 g carbohydrate, 25 g protein, 2.2 g total fat, less than 1 g saturated fat, 56 mg cholesterol, 152 mg sodium, 3.5 g dietary fiber, 9% calories from fat

CHICKEN BREAST WITH SHIITAKE MUSHROOM AND SUNDRIED TOMATO CREAM SAUCE

1 teaspoon garlic
1/2 cup diced onion
1/2 cup sliced sundried tomatoes
1/2 cup dry white wine
2 cups sliced button mushrooms
1 cup sliced shiitake mushrooms
1 teaspoon lemon juice
1/4 teaspoon dried thyme
1 tablespoon minced fresh basil
1 1/2 cups chicken broth
Pinch of black pepper
1 tablespoon low-sodium soy sauce
2 skinless chicken breasts (16 ounces)
1 teaspoon cornstarch dissolved in 2 tablespoons cold chicken broth
1/2 cup of Creamy Mixture

CREAMY MIXTURE

5 ounces evaporated skim milk
1/4 cup nonfat cream cheese
1 cup nonfat sour cream

Combine all ingredients in a food processor until creamy.

Simmer the garlic, onion, and sundried tomatoes for 2 minutes in the wine, covered.

Add the mushrooms, lemon juice, thyme, basil, chicken broth, pepper, soy sauce, and chicken breasts. Bring to a boil and cook for 7 minutes on medium heat, covered. Turn the chicken breasts over and cook for 7 minutes more. Remove the chicken breasts and thicken the sauce with the cornstarch mixture.

Add the creamy mixture and bring to a boil then lower the heat immediately. Do not allow the sauce to continue to boil once the creamy mixture has been added.

Serves 4

Per Serving: 268 calories, 14 g carbohydrate, 39 g protein, 3 g total fat, 84 mg cholesterol, 490 mg sodium, 2 g dietary fiber, 8% calories from fat

CHOCOLATE MOUSSE

10 ounces extra-firm lite silken tofu
1/4 cup evaporated skim milk
1/3 cup liquid Fruit Source® or Equal®
1/4 cup cocoa powder
1 1/2 teaspoons vanilla extract

Blend the tofu and milk until smooth.

Heat the Fruit Source® over low heat. Pour over the cocoa powder and whisk until smooth.

Pour the cocoa syrup and vanilla into the tofu and blend until smooth. Refrigerate for 4 hours.

Serves 5

Per serving: 94 calories, 11 g carbohydrate, 7 g protein, 2.6 g total fat, 0.16 g saturated fat, 0 mg cholesterol, 70 mg sodium, 0 g dietary fiber, 25% calories from fat

Note: Fruit Source® is a natural sweetener made from grains and grapes. It is available in natural foods stores in both liquid and granulated form, or call to order: 1-800-227-1577.

If using Equal®, just blend the cocoa powder, tofu, evaporated skim milk, and Equal® until smooth.

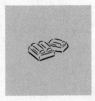

CLAM, LOBSTER, AND SEA SCALLOP PAELLA

1/2 teaspoon minced garlic
1/2 cup minced red bell pepper
1/2 cup minced red onion
1 cup diced carrots
1/2 cup white wine
1/2 cup clam juice
2 cups chopped tomatoes
1 tablespoon lemon juice
1/2 teaspoon curry powder
1/2 teaspoon paprika
Pinch of red pepper flakes
1/2 teaspoon fresh oregano
2 tablespoons chopped fresh basil
2 pounds fresh littleneck clams
3 lobster tails, cut into 1/2-inch pieces
1/2 pound large fresh scallops
1/2 cup cooked wild rice
3 cups cooked brown rice
1 cup frozen green peas
6 lemon wedges for garnish

In a large skillet, simmer the garlic, red pepper, onion, and diced carrots in the white wine and clam juice, covered, over medium heat for 5 minutes. Add the tomatoes, lemon juice, curry, paprika, red pepper flakes, and fresh herbs.

Add the clams, cook for 5 minutes, and remove the open clams. Cook for 5 minutes more, remove the open clams, and discard any clams that have not yet opened.

Add the lobster pieces, stir, and cook for 3 minutes. Add the scallops, rices, and peas and sauté, uncovered, for 5 minutes, stirring frequently.

Garnish with the steamed fresh clams and lemon wedges.

Serves 6

Per serving: 272 calories, 38 g carbohydrate, 21 g protein, 2 g total fat, 0.35 g saturated fat, 52 mg cholesterol, 244 mg sodium, 5 g dietary fiber, 8% calories from fat

COUNTRY MUSTARD VINAIGRETTE

1 tablespoon Grey Poupon Dijon Country mustard
3 tablespoons rice vinegar
1 teaspoon fresh lemon juice
1/4 teaspoon apple juice concentrate
1 cup sparkling water
Pinch of black pepper
1/8 teaspoon xantham gum (see Note)
3 tablespoons minced shallots

Blend all ingredients, except shallots, in an electric blender. Stir in the diced shallots and refrigerate, covered and dated, for no more than 10 days.

Note: Xantham gum is a natural thickener that can be found in health food stores.

Makes 2 cups

Per 2-tablespoon serving: 1.45 calories, less than 1 g carbohydrate, 0 g protein, 0 g fat, 0 mg cholesterol, 5 mg sodium

CRUNCHY TOFU AND ZUCCHINI BALLS

3 garlic cloves
1 large onion
2 cups shiitake mushrooms
1/2 cup chopped fresh parsley
1/4 cup chopped fresh basil
1/4 teaspoon dried thyme
1/4 teaspoon dried oregano
1 teaspoon diced jalapeño chili pepper
1 cup chopped green bell pepper
1 teaspoon low-sodium soy sauce
1 teaspoon balsamic vinegar
10 ounces Mori-Nu Lite extra-firm tofu, crumbled
2 cups shredded zucchini
1/4 cup egg whites
1/2 cup matzo meal

Preheat the oven to 325 degrees.

Spray a little olive oil or Pam in a medium skillet and sauté the garlic and onion over medium heat. Add the shiitake mushrooms, parsley, basil, thyme, oregano, peppers, and soy sauce. Sauté for 5 minutes more. Add the balsamic vinegar and stir while cooking for 1 minute more.

Transfer the mixture to a mixing bowl. Stir in the tofu, zucchini, egg whites, and matzo meal. Form into balls and bake on a greased baking sheet at 325 degrees for 30 minutes.

Serve over spaghetti squash with a spicy tomato sauce.

Serves 4

Per serving: 127 calories, 22 g carbohydrate, 8 g protein, 1 g fat, 0 g saturated fat, 0 mg cholesterol, 169 mg sodium, 2.5 g dietary fiber, 8% calories from fat

GREEN BEANS BARCELONA

1/2 cup vegetable broth
1/2 teaspoon minced garlic
1/2 cup chopped onion
1/2 cup red bell pepper, cut into thin strips
1/2 cup yellow bell pepper, cut into thin strips
1/8 teaspoon black pepper
1/2 teaspoon low-sodium soy sauce
3 cups cooked green beans
1/2 teaspoon minced fresh tarragon or basil
1 tablespoon chopped fresh parsley

In a large nonstick skillet, bring the broth to a boil and sauté the garlic, onion, and peppers for 5 minutes, covered, on medium heat.

Add the black pepper, soy sauce, and green beans. Simmer for 5 minutes, uncovered, stirring frequently. Garnish with fresh tarragon and parsley.

Serves 6

Per serving: 36 calories, 8 g carbohydrate, 1.89 g protein, 0 g total fat, 0 mg cholesterol, 33 mg sodium, 3 g dietary fiber

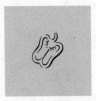

GREEN CABBAGE STEW

1 cup chopped onion
1/2 teaspoon minced garlic
3 cups shredded green cabbage
1 bay leaf
1/4 teaspoon cloves
2 tablespoons rice vinegar
1 1/2 teaspoons low-sodium soy sauce
1 tablespoon apple juice concentrate
1/4 teaspoon black pepper
Pinch of nutmeg
1/2 cup water
1/2 teaspoon cornstarch diluted in 1 tablespoon cold water (optional)

Spray a little olive oil or Pam in a large nonstick skillet and heat for 1 minute on medium heat. Sauté the onion and garlic, covered, on medium heat for 1 minute. Add the cabbage, bay leaf, cloves, rice vinegar, soy sauce, apple juice concentrate, black pepper, nutmeg, and water, cover, and cook for 20 minutes over medium heat.

Thicken with the cornstarch mixture if desired.

Serves 6

Per serving: 30 calories, 6.6 g carbohydrate, 1 g protein, 0 g total fat, 0 mg cholesterol, 56 mg sodium, 1.3 g dietary fiber

HUMMUS

---

    1 can (15 ounces) garbanzo beans, drained
    3 tablespoons lemon juice
    1 teaspoon minced garlic
    2 tablespoons nonfat sour cream
    1/4 cup fresh chopped parsley or cilantro
    Tabasco to taste
    1 teaspoon low-sodium soy sauce

Combine all ingredients in a food processor and blend until smooth and creamy.

Serves 8

Per serving: 97 calories, 16 g carbohydrate, 5 g protein, 1.5 g total fat, 0.1 g saturated fat, 0 mg cholesterol, 36 mg sodium, 4.4 g dietary fiber, 13% calories from fat

JUAN'S ROASTED GARLIC DIP

1 tablespoon minced roasted garlic
1½ cups cooked garbanzo beans
1 tablespoon lemon juice
1 teaspoon low-sodium soy sauce
¼ cup nonfat sour cream

Slowly roast a handful of unpeeled garlic cloves at 300 degrees until fully cooked (approximately 45 to 60 minutes). Peel and process in a food processor. Keep the roasted garlic refrigerated in a tightly closed jar.

Process all ingredients in a food processor until smooth and creamy.

Serves 6 to 10

Per serving: 117 calories, 20 g carbohydrate, 6 g protein, 2 g total fat, 0 g saturated fat, 0 mg cholesterol, 32 mg sodium, 5 g dietary fiber, 13% calories from fat

LENTIL SOUP

1 cup minced onion
1/2 teaspoon minced garlic
1/2 cup finely chopped celery
1/2 cup finely chopped leeks
1 cup diced carrots
1 1/2 cups dried lentils, rinsed
1 bay leaf
2 cloves
5 cups vegetable broth or cold water
2 teaspoons low-sodium soy sauce
1/2 teaspoon curry powder
Pinch of red pepper flakes
1 cup diced peeled potatoes
2 teaspoons salt-free tomato paste
2 teaspoons chopped fresh basil

Spray a little olive oil or Pam in a large soup pan and heat on medium heat for 1 minute. Sauté onion, garlic, celery, leeks, and carrots on medium heat for 5 minutes, stirring frequently.

Add the lentils, bay leaf, cloves, vegetable broth, soy sauce, curry powder, and red pepper flakes. Bring to a boil, lower the heat, and add the potatoes and the tomato paste dissolved in 1/2 cup hot water.

Simmer for 45 minutes, covered. Add the basil and serve.

Serves 6

Per serving: 108 calories, 20 g carbohydrate, 7.5 g protein, 0 g total fat, 0 mg cholesterol, 98 mg sodium, 8.5 g dietary fiber

MANGO RICE PUDDING

2 cups cooked brown rice
1 cinnamon stick
1 cup chopped mangoes
1 cup evaporated skim milk
1 tablespoon vanilla
¼ cup apple juice concentrate
2 tablespoons date sugar
6 fresh mint leaves

Combine the rice, cinnamon, mangoes, milk, vanilla, and apple juice concentrate in a large saucepan. Cook, uncovered, over low-medium heat for 10 minutes, stirring frequently.

Remove from the heat and let stand for 10 minutes, spoon into dessert dishes, and sprinkle with date sugar. Decorate with fresh mint leaves.

Serves 6

Per serving: 176 calories, 35 g carbohydrate, 5 g protein, 0 g total fat, 0 mg cholesterol, 56 mg sodium, 2.13 g dietary fiber

MEXICAN VEGETABLE SOUP WITH LIME AND CILANTRO

1 teaspoon minced garlic
1 cup minced red onion
1/2 teaspoon minced jalapeño chili pepper
1/2 cup red wine
1 cup diced carrots
1 cup green beans
2 cups chopped tomatoes
5 cups defatted chicken broth
1 cup Pritikin 3-bean chili
1/2 teaspoon cumin powder
1 tablespoon barbecue sauce
1 tablespoon low-sodium soy sauce
1 tablespoon minced fresh cilantro
1 tablespoon lime juice

Sauté the garlic, onion, and jalapeño in the wine for 3 minutes. Add the carrots, green beans, tomatoes, and chicken broth. Bring to a boil and cook for 20 minutes on medium heat, partially covered. Add the bean chili, cumin, barbecue sauce, soy sauce, cilantro, and lime juice. Simmer for 10 minutes.

Makes 10 cups

Per 1/2-cup serving: 95 calories, 16 g carbohydrate, 6 g protein, 0 g total fat, 0 g saturated fat, 0 mg cholesterol, 55 mg sodium, 0.8 g dietary fiber

MUSHROOM AND SPINACH SOUFFLÉ

1 teaspoon minced garlic
1 cup minced onion
2 cups sliced mushrooms
1/2 cup vegetable broth
6 cups drained cooked spinach
2 teaspoons lemon juice
2 teaspoons low-sodium soy sauce
1/4 teaspoon black pepper
2 cups whole wheat bread crumbs
2 cups nonfat ricotta cheese
4 egg whites

Spray a little olive oil or Pam on a large nonstick skillet. Heat the skillet for 1 minute on medium heat. Sauté the garlic and onion for 1 minute on medium heat. Add the mushrooms and cook for 4 minutes, covered, on high heat.

Add the broth, spinach, lemon juice, soy sauce, and pepper and sauté for 2 minutes, stirring frequently. Add the bread crumbs and ricotta cheese and blend in a food processor until smooth.

Beat the egg whites until foamy and fold into the spinach mixture. Spray 8 ramekins lightly with Pam and pour the spinach mixture into them. Bake, uncovered, in a preheated 350-degree oven for 20 minutes. Unmold and serve over tomato sauce.

Serves 8

Per serving: 180 calories, 25 g carbohydrate, 16 g protein, 2 g fat, 0.7 g saturated fat, 7 mg cholesterol, 260 mg sodium, 9% calories from fat

RED CABBAGE WITH APPLES AND CARAWAY SEEDS

1/2 cup red wine
1 cup chopped red onion
3 cups shredded red cabbage
1 bay leaf
2 tablespoons balsamic vinegar
1 1/2 teaspoons low-sodium soy sauce
1 tablespoon apple juice concentrate
1/2 teaspoon caraway seeds
1 Golden Delicious apple, peeled and sliced

In a large skillet, bring the wine to a boil and sauté the onion and red cabbage, covered, for 10 minutes on medium heat. Add the bay leaf, balsamic vinegar, soy sauce, apple juice concentrate, and caraway seeds. Cover with the sliced apples, reduce the heat to low, and cook for 25 minutes, covered, adding a little water if the cabbage becomes too dry.

Serves 6

Per serving: 59 calories, 11 g carbohydrate, 1 g protein, 0 g total fat, 0 mg cholesterol, 57 mg sodium, 1.6 g dietary fiber

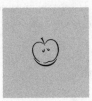

SALMON AND MUSHROOM RISOTTO

$1/2$ cup diced red pepper
$1/2$ cup diced onion
$1/2$ cup diced celery
2 cups sliced mushrooms
1 cup white wine
12 ounces fresh salmon fillet, skinned
1 cup clam juice
2 cups chopped tomatoes
$1/4$ cup cooked wild rice
$1 1/2$ cups cooked brown rice
1 teaspoon curry powder
Black pepper to taste
1 tablespoon lemon juice
2 tablespoons minced fresh parsley

In a large skillet, simmer the red pepper, onion, celery, and mushrooms for 10 minutes, covered, over medium heat in the white wine. Add the salmon, clam juice, tomatoes, cooked rices, curry powder, and black pepper.

Cook, uncovered, over low heat, stirring, until most of the liquid is absorbed, about 7 minutes. Add the lemon juice and parsley and serve.

Serves 4

Per serving: 305 calories, 31 g carbohydrate, 21 g protein, 7 g fat, 1 g saturated fat, 46 mg cholesterol, 207 mg sodium, 4.6 g dietary fiber, 20% calories from fat

SEA BASS WITH ASPARAGUS CREAM SAUCE

1/2 cup minced shallots
1/2 cup dry white wine
Pinch of black pepper
2 tablespoons white wine Worcestershire sauce
1 1/2 cups chicken or vegetable broth
3 cups chopped asparagus
1 pound Chilean sea bass
1 teaspoon lemon juice
1 teaspoon cornstarch dissolved in 2 tablespoons cold chicken broth
1/2 cup Creamy Mixture (page 222)
2 tablespoons minced fresh dill or parsley

Sauté the shallots in the wine for 1 minute. Add the pepper, Worcestershire sauce, broth, asparagus, sea bass, and lemon juice. Bring to a boil and cook for 5 minutes on medium heat, covered. Turn the sea bass upside down and cook for 5 minutes more.

Remove the sea bass, thicken the sauce with the cornstarch mixture, and add the creamy mixture to the sauce; bring to a boil then lower heat immediately.

Blend the sauce in a food processor, pour the sauce over the sea bass, and sprinkle with the dill.

Serves 4

Per serving: 240 calories, 13 g carbohydrate, 33 g protein, 3 g total fat, 0.8 g saturated fat, 274 mg sodium, 2.5 g dietary fiber, 11% calories from fat

SHIITAKE MUSHROOM STROGANOFF

15 ounces Mori-Nu Lite silken tofu
2 tablespoons low-sodium soy sauce
1 teaspoon minced garlic
$1/2$ cup diced onion
$1/2$ cup sliced sundried tomatoes
$1/2$ cup dry white wine
2 cups sliced mushrooms
1 cup sliced shiitake mushrooms
1 teaspoon lemon juice
$1/4$ teaspoon dried thyme
1 tablespoon minced fresh basil
$11/2$ cups chicken broth
Pinch of black pepper
1 teaspoon cornstarch dissolved in 2 tablespoons cold chicken broth
$1/2$ cup Creamy Mixture (page 222)

Cut the tofu into $1/2$-inch cubes and marinate in the soy sauce for 30 minutes, refrigerated.

In a large skillet, over medium-low heat, sauté the garlic, onion, and sundried tomatoes for 2 minutes in the wine. Add the mushrooms, lemon juice, thyme, basil, broth, and pepper. Bring to a boil and cook for 5 minutes on medium heat, covered.

Add the tofu cubes and soy sauce marinade. Cook for 5 more minutes, uncovered. Thicken the sauce with the cornstarch mixture. Add the creamy mixture and bring to a boil, then lower the heat and immediately add the basil.

Serves 4

Per serving: 162 calories, 20 g carbohydrate, 15 g protein, 3 g total fat, 0.34 g saturated fat, 2 mg cholesterol, 317 mg sodium, 2.5 g dietary fiber, 15% calories from fat

SOUPE AU PISTOU (NIÇOISE VEGETABLE SOUP)

---

1 cup small white beans
1 cup diced onion
2 cups diced leeks
2 tablespoons minced garlic
4 quarts water
2 cups diced zucchini
2 cups shredded cabbage
2 cups diced banana squash
2 cups diced potatoes
2 cups green beans
2 cups diced carrots
1 teaspoon dried thyme
1 bay leaf
1/4 teaspoon dried sage
3 tablespoons white wine Worcestershire sauce
Pinch of black pepper
1 cup cooked lima beans
1 cup uncooked macaroni
4 tablespoons balsamic vinegar
4 tablespoons fresh basil

Bring the beans to a boil in enough water to cover and cook over medium heat for 10 minutes. Drain and rinse the beans thoroughly.

Sauté the onion, leeks, and garlic in 1/2 cup water for 5 minutes. Add all vegetables, the beans, and the remaining water. Add the thyme, bay leaf, sage, Worcestershire sauce, and black pepper. Bring to a boil and simmer, covered, for 40 minutes.

Add the lima beans and macaroni and simmer for 15 minutes. Add the vinegar and fresh basil.

Serves 15

Per serving: 105 calories, 22 g carbohydrate, 5 g protein, 0 g total fat, 0 mg cholesterol, 100 mg sodium, 4 g dietary fiber

STUFFED POTATOES

4 baked potatoes
1/2 cup nonfat sour cream
2 tablespoons skim milk
1 tablespoon chopped fresh parsley
Pinch of white pepper
Pinch of nutmeg

Slice the baked potatoes in halves. With a teaspoon, remove the potato pulp and set the empty skins aside.

Puree the pulp and add the sour cream, milk, parsley, pepper, and nutmeg. Blend as you would mashed potatoes. Fill the potato skins with the potato mixture and bake, uncovered, for 10 minutes at 350 degrees.

Serves 4

Per serving: 261 calories, 58 g carbohydrate, 7 g protein, 0 g total fat, 0 mg cholesterol, 46 mg sodium, 5 g dietary fiber

SPINACH ROLL-UPS

2 cups fat-free sour cream
1 tablespoon low-sodium soy sauce
$1/4$ teaspoon garlic powder
$1/4$ teaspoon onion powder
$1/8$ teaspoon black pepper
$1 1/2$ cups cooked spinach, drained
1 package soft, whole wheat lavash bread

In a food processor, blend the sour cream, soy sauce, garlic powder, onion powder, and black pepper until smooth. Add the drained spinach and blend a little more so that the spinach is distributed but not completely blended.

Spread the spinach mixture evenly over the lavash bread. Roll up and refrigerate for several hours. When ready to serve, slice into pinwheels.

Serves 10

Per serving: 102 calories, 19 g carbohydrate, 5.8 g protein, 0 g total fat, 0 mg cholesterol, 219 mg sodium, 3 g dietary fiber

SZECHUAN TOFU AND FRIED RICE

2 packages (20 ounces) Mori-Nu extra-firm tofu
2 tablespoons lite soy sauce
$1/3$ cup pineapple juice
3 tablespoons sugar-free raspberry preserves
$1^1/_2$ tablespoons rice vinegar
Pinch of crushed red pepper
$1^1/_2$ tablespoons lemon juice
1 teaspoon minced garlic
2 teaspoons minced ginger
$1/3$ cup water
$1/_2$ teaspoon chili powder
$1/_2$ teaspoon sweet basil
$1/_2$ teaspoon curry powder

The day before, slice each piece of tofu into $3/_4$-inch cubes. Lay the cubes of tofu on a baking tray and cover with plastic wrap. Freeze overnight.

The next day, put the frozen tofu cubes into boiling water to thaw. Place the tofu cubes in an 11 × 7-inch baking dish. Combine the remaining ingredients and pour over the tofu. Bake at 400 degrees, uncovered, for 15 minutes.

FRIED RICE

1 teaspoon minced garlic
$1/4$ cup minced onion
2 tablespoons dry sherry
2 tablespoons water
Pinch of black pepper
2 cups cooked brown rice
1 cup green peas
1 cup frozen corn kernels

On high heat, sauté the garlic and onion in the sherry until the wine is evaporated. Add the water, pepper, and warm cooked rice. Stir in the peas and corn. Cook until heated through.

Serves 6

Per serving: 218 calories, 35 g carbohydrate, 12 g protein, 2 g total fat, 0 g saturated fat, 0 mg cholesterol, 302 mg sodium, 2.5 g dietary fiber

TUNA SALAD

1 tablespoon Grey Poupon mustard
1 tablespoon Kozlowski's hot and sweet mustard
Black pepper or Tabasco to taste
1 tablespoon lemon juice
1 cup nonfat sour cream
8 ounces water-packed tuna
1 cup minced carrots
1/2 cup minced bell pepper
1/2 cup minced onion
1 cup minced celery
1/4 cup minced fresh dill or parsley

Add the mustards, pepper, and lemon juice to the sour cream. Add the remaining ingredients and mix well.

Serves 6

Per serving: 91 calories, 13 g carbohydrate, 7 g protein, 0 g total fat, 4.5 mg cholesterol, 94 mg sodium, 1.5 g dietary fiber

TURKEY BREAST MEAT LOAF

1½ pounds ground turkey breast
1 cup minced onion
1 tablespoon minced garlic
1 cup minced carrots
½ cup minced celery
½ cup minced parsley
1 cup oatmeal
1 cup bread crumbs
3 tablespoons salt-free tomato paste
3 tablespoons salt-free Dijon mustard
3 tablespoons Worcestershire sauce
½ cup barbecue sauce
1 teaspoon dried thyme
¼ teaspoon black pepper
4 egg whites
Tabasco to taste
½ cup salt-free tomato sauce

In a mixing bowl, combine all ingredients, except the tomato sauce, until well mixed. Spray the meat loaf pan with nonstick cooking spray.

Pour the turkey mixture into the meat loaf pan (approximately 8 inches by 4 inches) and bake for 45 minutes, covered, at 375 degrees. Pour the tomato sauce over the meat loaf and bake for 25 minutes, uncovered, at 375 degrees.

Remove the meat loaf from the oven, and let it sit for 20 minutes before slicing.

Serves 8

Per serving: 330 calories, 31 g carbohydrate, 25 g protein, 5 g total fat, 3 g saturated fat, 69 mg cholesterol, 269 mg sodium, 5 g dietary fiber, 14 % total calories from fat

VEGETABLE COUSCOUS

1 onion, diced
3 garlic cloves, minced
1 green bell pepper, sliced
2 diced carrots
2 leeks, chopped
2 celery stalks, chopped
1 15-ounce can chickpeas, rinsed and drained
1 bay leaf
1 fresh jalapeño chili pepper, seeded and chopped
1 can (28 ounces) chopped tomatoes
2 quarts cold water
3 turnips, peeled and quartered
1/2 teaspoon saffron threads
2 tablespoons low-sodium soy sauce
4 zucchini, sliced
1 bunch cilantro or Italian parsley, chopped
1 pound couscous
Lemon wedges for garnish

Spray the bottom of a large heavy-bottomed pot with a little olive oil or Pam. Over medium heat, simmer the onion, garlic, green pepper, carrots, leeks, and celery for 5 minutes, covered, stirring a few times.

Add the chickpeas, bay leaf, jalapeño pepper, and tomatoes and simmer for 10 minutes, covered.

Add the water, turnips, saffron threads, and soy sauce. Bring to a boil and simmer for 30 minutes. Add the zucchini and cilantro and simmer 15 minutes longer.

Thirty minutes before you wish to serve the dish, place the couscous in a large bowl and gradually sprinkle on about 2 cups of water. Let it sit for 15 minutes, stirring between your palms and fingers every 5 minutes to prevent the couscous from lumping.

Bring the soup back to a simmer.

To serve, spoon the couscous into large soup bowls and ladle a generous serving of the soup on top. Garnish with lemon wedges.

Serves 12

Per serving: 262 calories, 52 g carbohydrate, 1.5 g total fat, 0 mg cholesterol, 173 mg sodium, 4.5 dietary fiber, 5 % calories from fat

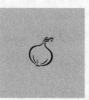

VEGETARIAN MEAT LOAF

16 Pritikin or Boca burgers, thawed
1½ 16-ounce can garbanzo beans, drained and chopped
1 cup chopped red peppers
1 cup chopped onion
2 teaspoons minced garlic
3 tablespoons chopped fresh basil
½ cup chopped fresh parsley
1 cup chopped green bell pepper
¼ cup egg whites
½ cup plus 2 tablespoons salt-free, sugar-free barbecue sauce

Process the Pritikin or Boca burgers and the beans in a food processor. In a mixing bowl, combine the remaining ingredients, except 2 tablespoons of barbecue sauce. Add the burger mixture and mix well.

Place the burger mixture in a loaf pan and bake at 400 degrees, covered, for 30 minutes. Top with an additional 2 tablespoons barbecue sauce and bake, uncovered, for an additional 15 minutes.

Serves 10 to 12

Per serving: 125 calories, 16 g carbohydrate, 14 g protein, 0 g total fat, 0 mg cholesterol, 255 mg sodium, 7 g dietary fiber, 0% from fat

WHITE BEANS AND TOMATO SOUP WITH PARSLEY PESTO

1/2 cup dry navy beans
1/2 teaspoon minced garlic
1/2 cup minced red onion
1/2 teaspoon minced jalapeño chili pepper
1/2 cup white wine
1 cup diced carrots
1 bay leaf
1/2 teaspoon dried thyme
1 tablespoon low-sodium soy sauce
1/2 teaspoon chili powder
1/2 teaspoon ground cumin
8 cups cold water
1 tablespoon salt-free tomato paste
2 cups chopped peeled tomatoes
1 tablespoon balsamic vinegar
8 teaspoons parsley pesto (recipe follows)

Rinse the navy beans and place in a large soup pan. Cover with cold water, cover the pan, and bring to a boil. Lower the heat and simmer for 10 minutes. Drain the beans and rinse thoroughly.

In a large soup pan, sauté the garlic, onion, and jalapeño in the wine, over medium heat for 2 minutes. Add the carrots, rinsed beans, bay leaf, thyme, soy sauce, chili powder, cumin, and 7 cups of cold water. Bring to a boil, lower the heat to low, and simmer for 45 minutes, covered. Dissolve the tomato paste in the remaining 1 cup of water and add to the soup with the chopped tomatoes and balsamic vinegar. Simmer for 15 minutes.

Serve the soup in bowls and top each with 1 teaspoon parsley pesto.

Serves 8

Per serving: 83 calories, 14 g carbohydrate, 4 g protein, 0 g total fat, 0 mg cholesterol, 98 mg sodium, 4.6 g dietary fiber

PARSLEY PESTO

1/2 cup chopped fresh parsley
1/4 cup nonfat sour cream
1/2 teaspoon minced garlic
1/4 cup cooked garbanzo beans
1 tablespoon lemon juice
1 teaspoon low-sodium soy sauce
1 teaspoon Dijon mustard
Pinch of black pepper

Blend all ingredients in a food processor and keep refrigerated.

Makes 1 cup of pesto

Per serving: 35 calories, 6 g carbohydrate, 2 g protein, 0 g total fat, 0 mg cholesterol, 37 mg sodium, 1.2 g dietary fiber

APPENDIX

All the information and the dietary guidelines I provide throughout *The Pritikin Weight Loss Breakthrough* apply primarily to people concerned with weight loss, those who want to improve their health, and those who wish to avoid the major degenerative diseases, including heart disease, high blood pressure, overweight, and several types of cancer. They are also applicable to those with adult-onset (type II) diabetes. If you fall within those groups, the program described in chapter 7 is designed for you.

There are, however, two acute conditions for which small but significant modifications should be made to the Pritikin Program: coronary heart disease (and specifically its underlying cause, atherosclerosis) and high blood pressure (also referred to as hypertension). There are also some people who adopt the Pritikin Program to help overcome serious illness, but in the course of following our eating plan find that they are losing more weight than they desire. While there is no threat to health from weight loss associated with the Pritikin Program, some people nonetheless prefer to be a little heavier than the weight they achieve. Only small changes are required on the Pritikin Program to help you speed recovery from coronary artery disease or high blood pressure or achieve a weight that is more comfortable for you.

FOR PEOPLE WHO ALREADY SUFFER FROM ATHEROSCLEROSIS

Atherosclerosis is the formation of cholesterol plaques that arise like boils within arteries, especially within the coronary arteries that bring blood and oxygen to the heart. These plaques are the underlying cause of most heart attacks and strokes.

Atherosclerosis strikes when blood cholesterol levels become excessive. For the vast majority of people, the two most important factors that contribute to high blood cholesterol levels are foods rich in saturated fats and cholesterol. Other important factors are cigarette smoking and diabetes. The heart disease rates of diabetics are three times those of non-diabetics. Their elevated insulin levels and overweight combine to promote the creation of atherosclerotic plaques.

The Mechanics of High Cholesterol

We consume three types of fats from our diet: saturated fats, which are found mostly in animal products such as red meat, chicken, eggs, and fish; polyunsaturated fats, derived mostly from vegetables and from cold water fish such as salmon, mackerel, and sardines; and monounsaturated fats, which are found most commonly in olives, olive oil, and canola oil. Of these three, only saturated fats will raise your blood cholesterol, though all three types of fats will increase your weight.

All plant foods contain some fat, though most contain only small amounts of it. These fats can be extracted from plants as oils. Research has shown that polyunsaturated oils lower blood cholesterol somewhat, but diets that contain too many polyunsaturated oils are suspected of contributing cancer. They can also lower your high density lipoproteins (HDL), or the so-called good cholesterol that protects against heart disease. Monounsaturated fats have little independent effect on cholesterol and are not associated with cancer, but they will increase weight. Monounsaturated fats can contribute to a lower blood cholesterol level if they replace saturated fats in your diet, however.

Cholesterol is obtained only from animal foods; there is no cholesterol in vegetables, or in vegetable oils. Animal foods, therefore, contain both saturated fats and cholesterol.

When saturated fats and cholesterol are consumed, the liver is stimulated to produce more cholesterol. At the same time, the liver's ability to remove cholesterol from the blood is impaired, as well. These factors combine to increase the amount of cholesterol in the blood.

Both cholesterol and saturated fat are carried inside the blood as packages, or complexes called lipoproteins. After a series of refinements, those packages of protein and cholesterol become low-density lipoproteins (LDL), the type of cholesterol that, in elevated amounts, causes atherosclerosis, heart disease, and stroke.

After it enters the bloodstream, LDL particles can sink into the wall of the artery, where they can undergo a chemical change, called oxidation. Essentially, they decay, or break down, just as metal does when it rusts, or when an apple decays and browns. Because oxidation can disrupt chemical processes within the cell, the oxidized LDL is recognized by the body as a threat to health. Immune cells rush to the area and consume the decaying LDL particles, and in the process become engorged with oxidized cholesterol. As more and more engorged immune cells collect within the wall of the artery, they form what is called a fatty streak. This is the first stage of atherosclerosis. If sufficient saturated fat and cholesterol continue to be consumed, the fatty streak will grow larger until it becomes a full-blown plaque.

The Dangers of Atherosclerotic Plaques

For decades, scientists believed that heart attacks were caused when these plaques became so large that they completely walled off one or more of the arteries to the heart, stopping blood flow and causing part of the heart to suffocate and die. The death of part of the heart muscle is called a *myocardial infarction* or a heart attack.

Actually, only a minority of heart attacks are caused when the arteries are sealed off in this way. Most heart attacks are caused by plaques that are relatively small and, by themselves, are not at all large enough to cut off blood flow to the heart. Unfortunately, these small plaques have a way of growing rapidly and causing big trouble.

Most plaques have a hard, fibrous surface called a cap, but inside the plaques are highly unstable pools of viscous cholesterol and fat. These plaques look very like a swollen, pus-filled pimple within the artery. Unstable plaques can erupt and burst open, causing an open wound in the artery wall. As with any wound in the body, clotting proteins and blood platelets collect over the rupture, forming a blood clot, or *thrombus*. Unlike the fibrous cap, the blood clot is also unstable, especially since it sits atop an open wound. Blood that contains high amounts of cholesterol can actually increase the fluid content within the plaques, causing the fibrous cap to be stretched and broken. This makes the plaque highly unstable and increases the likelihood that it will rupture. As more plaques rupture, the more blood clots form within the arteries. Many other factors are involved to make the plaque more unstable, including clotting proteins and blood platelets, which become sticky from a high-fat diet and increase the likelihood of forming clots.

In the process of closing off an open wound within the vessel, these blood blots can become so large that they themselves can block blood flow to the heart muscle, and thereby suffocate the heart and bring on a heart attack. Most heart attacks are caused by the formation of a blood clot that blocks blood flow to the heart, a process called *coronary thrombosis*.

Many strokes are caused in the same way: a clot blocks blood from flowing to the brain. Once blood flow to a part of the brain is impeded or stopped, those tissues of the brain can suffocate and die, causing a stroke.

The pool of viscous cholesterol at the center of the plaque, the presence of high levels of cholesterol within the blood, and the tendency of blood constituents to form clots all combine to make atherosclerotic plaques highly unstable and likely to rupture. Once the plaque opens and clots begin to form, the risk of suffering a heart attack or stroke dramatically increases.

This understanding has revolutionized the scientific approach to coronary heart disease. Scientists no longer believe that reversal of the atherosclerotic plaque, which takes years to accomplish, is necessary to take people out of acute danger; instead, they emphasize the stabilization of the atherosclerotic plaque. If you stop a plaque from rupturing, you can prevent coronary thrombosis.

How to Lower Blood Cholesterol

The key to stabilizing the plaques and preventing heart attacks is to eat a diet that will lower blood cholesterol and other blood constituents, and reduce the tendency of blood to form clots. This will prevent plaques from swelling, breaking open, and forming a thrombosis.

Blood cholesterol levels can fall dramatically within one month. The evidence suggests that within 30 days of adopting the Pritikin diet, plaques can be stabilized and your chances of suffering a heart attacked reduced substantially. In effect, you can take yourself out of acute danger of having a heart attack simply by following the Pritikin Program for several weeks. On the other hand, eating just a few high-fat meals can reverse any progress you made, and put you back in danger of rupturing plaques.

Many factors will lower cholesterol levels, but the most important one is to significantly reduce or eliminate saturated fats and cholesterol from your diet. If you have advanced coronary heart disease, I recommend that you sharply reduce your intake of saturated fat, cholesterol, and animal protein. As a result, your blood cholesterol will fall dramatically. The sharp reduction of dietary fats also reduces clotting proteins and prevents blood platelets from sticking together and helping to form clots.

People with advanced coronary disease should eat only two servings per day of nonfat dairy products. In addition, they should eat only $3^{1}/_{2}$ to 7 ounces of cold-water fish such as salmon, mackerel, or sardines once a week. These fish contain a type of polyunsaturated fat called omega-3, which has been shown to reduce the tendency of blood to form clots. No other animal foods should be eaten.

Several other factors can lower blood cholesterol and reduce your risk of heart attack and stroke. Soluble fibers found in beans, soybeans, oats, barley, citrus fruits, apples, pears, and root vegetables have been shown to bind with fat and cholesterol in the intestinal tract and eliminate it from the body, thereby lowering overall blood cholesterol. Beans and soybean products have been shown to be especially potent at lowering blood cholesterol because of their soluble fibers as well as their relatively high vegetable-protein content, which independently lowers blood cholesterol. Animal protein, by contrast, increases blood cholesterol levels. Plants also contain fiber-based sterols that may lower blood cholesterol.

Meal frequency also influences blood cholesterol levels. Studies have shown that when the same foods are eaten more frequently throughout the course of the day, blood cholesterol levels are lowered by 8 to 15 percent. As you know, eating frequently is one of the pillars of the Pritikin Program.

In addition to encouraging you to eat a plant-based diet, the Pritikin Program also recommends daily exercise, which for most people need be only a daily walk. Walking is ideal for people with coronary disease because it does not overstress the heart but nonetheless exercises the heart muscle and improves circulation. Exercise can lower triglycerides and blood pressure. It also has the tendency to raise HDL cholesterol.

Finally, research has shown that vitamin E reduces the blood's tendency to form clots. As an antioxidant, it also prevents the oxidation of some of the LDL particles, thereby shutting down the first step in the formation of atherosclerosis. Physicians at the Pritikin Longevity Center recommend a daily dosage of 400 international units of vitamin E for those at risk.

In addition to vitamin E, I also recommend that you talk to your doctor about taking aspirin to reduce the blood's tendency to form clots. You should not take aspirin on any sort of regular basis without talking to your physician first, however. Aspirin can cause harmful side effects in some people.

As I reported in chapter 2, researchers at the Pritikin Longevity Center have demonstrated a significant drop in the average blood cholesterol and triglyceride levels among people who come to our centers and adopt our program. The average drop in cholesterol is 23 percent; the average drop in trigylycerides, or blood fats, is 33 percent.

We've also had a remarkable track record when it comes to restoring type II or adult-onset diabetics to normal function, not only reducing their symptoms, but also preventing the disorders that often accompany diabetes, such as blindness, heart attack, claudication, and amputation of limbs due to poor circulation and gangrene. Thirty-nine percent of people who come to our center taking insulin leave insulin-free. Of the adult-onset diabetics who came to our center taking oral medication, 70 percent no longer needed their diabetes drugs when they leave.

SUMMARY OF RECOMMENDATIONS TO TREAT ATHEROSCLEROSIS

The following recommendations will have a dramatic effect on atherosclerosis, and significantly reduce your risk of suffering a heart attack or stroke:

- Reduce fat, cholesterol, and animal proteins by eating only two servings of nonfat dairy products per day, and only $3^1/_2$ to 7 ounces of cold-water fish per week. The recommended fish are salmon, mackerel, and sardines. These fish contain omega-3 polyunsaturated fats that reduce the blood's tendency to form clots.

- Eliminate all other animal foods, including red meats, chicken, eggs, and whole-milk products such as cheese.

- Make the vast majority of your foods plant-based to increase soluble fibers, vegetable proteins, and plant sterols.

- Eat frequently. In addition to your three main meals per day, eat three healthful snacks. (See chapters 6 and 7 for specific recommendations on meal frequency, menu ideas, and recommended snacks.)

- Walk daily to lower triglycerides, reduce blood pressure, and increase HDL levels.

- Talk to your doctor about taking aspirin and 400 IU of vitamin E daily.

FOR PEOPLE WITH HIGH BLOOD PRESSURE

Several lifestyle-related factors increase your chance of suffering from high blood pressure, also known as hypertension, but one of the most important of these is the excess consumption of salt, or sodium chloride. Scientists used to believe that it was just the sodium in the salt that raised blood pressure, but new evidence has revealed that it is the combination of both sodium and chloride—or regular salt—that can cause elevations in blood pressure.

Blood pressure is considered high when the top number is 140 and higher, and the bottom number is 90 and higher. For generations, scientists believed that high blood pressure was an inevitable by-product of aging, but then they discovered many populations who aged without ever becoming hypertensive. Not surprisingly, the populations who did not develop hypertension were those who remained on their traditional low-sodium diets. Those populations of peoples whose traditional diets are high in salt, such as the Japanese and Chinese, have higher levels of hypertension—even though these peoples typically eat diets very low in fat and refined foods. Studies have shown that the protection of low-salt diets does not travel with people when they move to the West and adopt more westernized eating patterns. Like those who live in the Western world, traditional people who adopt a Western diet get hypertension just like the rest of us.

The Role of Salt

The vast majority of us enjoy and prefer salty foods. This is ironic, and even a bit peculiar, since there is no nutritional need for us to add salt to our food. Our kidneys are exquisitely designed to retain salt. Even if your diet is extremely low in salt, your kidneys will retain almost all the salt that passes through them; your body can effectively regulate the amount of salt in its tissues. Moreover, salt is plentiful in a wide variety of foods.

As omnivores, humans have evolved on diets that included animal foods, which contain salt. Also, it seems unlikely that we experienced extended periods of salt deprivation, which—had they occurred—would have caused us to develop a salt instinct much like our fat instinct.

Scientists speculate that our preference for salty foods may have arisen from two sources, one very ancient, the other modern. It may be that one of our ancestors subsisted entirely on fruit and vegetables, which would have provided small amounts of salt, thus giving rise to a preference for salty foods in order to maintain adequate salt levels. It's possible that a vestige of that preference for salt may still be with us.

On the other hand, scientists have found that infants have no preference for salty-tasting foods. Salt was put into baby food because mothers thought that their babies would like the taste better, as they themselves did when they sampled the salted and unsalted baby foods. Also, research has shown that adults who consistently avoid salt experience a diminution in their preference for salty flavored foods. All of this has led some scientists to believe that our preference for salt is not an instinctual, but a learned behavior.

Still, our preference for salty foods, no matter whether it is learned or instinctual, is a powerful force in our food choices. Most authoritative sources recommend that you eat a minimum of 500 mg of salt per day. Food labels list the sodium content of the food, as opposed to the "salt" content. Since sodium is only part of salt, the recommended 500 mg. of salt per day translates as only 200 mg. of sodium each day. A "sodium-free" food contains less than 5 mg of sodium. A "very low sodium" food contains 35 mg of sodium per serving, while a "low-sodium" food contains 140 mg per serving. You can see that two servings of a "low-sodium" food will put you over the daily minimum recommended for sodium.

Excess consumption of salt depletes calcium levels from bones and leads to high rates of osteoporosis, or porous bones. By causing the excretion of calcium from bones, high-salt diets also increase the amount of calcium in the bloodstream and in the kidneys, which, in turn, increases the likelihood of kidney stones.

Other Factors Affecting High Blood Pressure

Other factors that contribute to high blood pressure include high-fat diets, overweight, excess alcohol consumption, and diets low in calcium, potassium, and magnesium.

Outside of diet, the most important lifestyle factor affecting blood pressure is exercising. Daily exercise appears to lower blood pressure.

At the Pritikin Longevity Center we have had significant success in reducing blood pressure and taking people off their medication. Of those studied who came to our center with high blood pressure and taking medication, 83 percent left with normal blood pressure and free of any need for pharmaceutical drugs.

SUMMARY OF RECOMMENDATIONS TO TREAT HIGH BLOOD PRESSURE

The following recommendations will dramatically reduce your risk of developing high blood pressure. If you already have hypertension, these recommendations will either prevent it from getting worse or help you to overcome it.

- Reduce or eliminate foods that contain salt or moderate to high amounts of salt, and avoid using salt as a condiment or in cooking.

- Use products that are salt-free or contain very low salt.

- Sharply reduce fat and cholesterol by following the Pritikin Program outlined in chapter 7.

- Eat foods rich in calcium, such as dark green vegetables and nonfat dairy products.

- Eat foods rich in potassium and magnesium, such as fruits, vegetables, and whole grains. The Pritikin Eating Plan provides an abundance of foods rich in potassium and magnesium.

- Exercise daily.

FOR PEOPLE WHO FEEL THAT THEY ARE LOSING TOO MUCH WEIGHT ON THE PRITIKIN PROGRAM

As many normal-weight people have found, a slim body does not guarantee freedom from heart disease or high blood pressure. Many people of normal weight have dangerously high blood cholesterol levels and coronary artery disease; others have high blood pressure. For all of these reasons, many lean people adopt the Pritikin Program.

We also attract many healthy athletes who want to maximize energy on a high carbohydrate diet, or avoid excess body fat that might reduce athletic performance. Our program accomplishes both of these goals, just as it prevents disease and helps people restore their health.

Still, people of low-to-normal weight who adopt the Pritikin Program inevitably experience some weight loss. Most of that lost weight comes from the shedding of body fat, which means that these people are healthier on our eating plan, but sometimes thinner than they want to be.

If you are such a person, the first thing you must realize is that being underweight is associated with longevity. Research has shown that men who are 20 percent below the average weight for Americans in their age group have a longer life expectancy than those who are at or above the national average. This is probably the case with women, as well.

Having said that, I acknowledge that from time to time, I meet people who tell me that they enjoy the diet and have experienced tremendous results on the Program, but would like to gain a little weight. "I've got good energy and I feel great, but I'd just like a few more pounds on me," they say. If you are among such people, here are my suggestions.

How to Gain Weight on the Pritikin Program

The first thing we recommend is that you increase concentrated sources of carbohydrates, such as breads, all-fruit jams, dried fruit, dry cereals, and fat-free chips. This step alone is often an effective way to stop weight loss and add a few pounds to those who are thin. On the other hand, some people who increase these foods significantly may experience a drop in HDL cholesterol and an elevation in triglycerides and insulin levels. This occurs especially in people who do not exercise. Exercise tends to protect people against elevations in triglycerides.

Because of the possibility of elevating triglycerides, diabetics should not increase fruit, all-fruit jams, dried cereals, and fat-free chips. Elevated triglycerides raise insulin levels and reduce insulin sensitivity—two factors that increase the risk of heart disease, blindness, poor circulation, and other dangerous conditions related to diabetes.

One way to combat such adverse effects is to increase exercise, particularly weight training, which will add muscle to your body. Muscle is dense and heavy tissue. It will add weight to your body without adding fat. By combining the exercise recommendations I have given, you can burn fat and lose weight from the aerobic exercise, while you increase muscle mass with the weight training. In the process, you may lose ten pounds of fat and add ten pounds of muscle. The scale will tell you that nothing has happened, but one look in the mirror will tell you otherwise. As I have said, exercise lowers triglycerides and blood pressure and also has the tendency to raise blood levels of HDL.

An effective weight training program can consist of twenty to thirty minutes of exercise, two to three times per week. People with coronary heart disease should consult their physicians before taking up such a program, however.

For the Lean Person with High Cholesterol and/or Hypertension

For the thin person with a high cholesterol level and a family history of heart disease, eating vegetable foods with higher mono- and polyunsaturated fat contents could increase your weight without boosting your cholesterol level. Moderate amounts of nuts and seeds may actually reduce your risk of heart attack and lower your blood cholesterol level, especially if they are eaten instead of animal foods, such as red meat, chicken, and eggs (all of which contain saturated fat and cholesterol).

Eating small amounts of avocados and including monounsaturated oils, such as olive, canola, and hazelnut in your diet will either add weight, or reduce the loss of body fat.

Nut butters—peanut, sesame, and almond—can be added in moderation to the diets of lean people who do not suffer from coronary artery disease or high blood pressure. They should be used sparingly, however, because they increase blood clotting and therefore increase

he risk of heart attack and stroke. Nut butters that have been hydro-
enated, or converted into saturated fats, should be avoided entirely,
specially by people with coronary heart disease and/or hypertension.

As avocados and vegetable oils do not contain salt (unless added)
mall amounts would be acceptable to thin people with high blood
ressure. Use these foods moderately; do not use them to increase
our weight. Weight gain would only increase your hypertension and
ut you at greater risk of suffering a heart attack or stroke.

People with high blood pressure but healthy cholesterol levels may
ncrease their intake of cold-water fish. This will elevate the fat con-
ent of their diets, without driving saturated fat levels up significantly.
The higher polyunsaturated fat content may reduce the likelihood of
lood clotting, and may help lower blood pressure as well.

The Pritikin Program recommends that you eat at least four serv-
ngs of vegetable foods and at least three servings of fruit per day. Very
ften, people snack on raw vegetables and other high-satiety, low-
alorie foods, thus boosting the number of high-satiety servings per
lay. Eating these foods will cause accelerated weight loss. Therefore,
imiting high-satiety, low-calorie foods to the minimum recom-
nended amounts each day and supplementing the eating plan with
he higher-calorie foods mentioned above will either slow weight loss,
top it, or add weight.

Finally, lean people should not overeat or force-feed themselves
ust to gain weight. This will only increase triglyceride levels, reduce
HDL, and increase your likelihood of heart disease. Don't compro-
nise your health to gain weight. There are lots of things you can do to
afely stabilize your weight.

SUMMARY OF RECOMMENDATIONS FOR LEAN PEOPLE WHO WANT TO GAIN WEIGHT

■ Increase concentrated sources of carbohydrates, such as breads, all-
   fruit jams, dried fruit, dry cereals, and fat-free chips. If you have
   coronary heart disease, be sure to monitor your triglycerides and
   HDL levels.

■ Increase exercise, both aerobic exercise and weight training. In addition to twenty minutes of daily aerobic exercise, such as walking, do twenty to thirty minutes of weight training, two to three times per week. This will increase muscle mass.

■ Lean people with high cholesterol levels should increase their intake of vegetable foods with higher mono- and polyunsaturated fat contents, such as nuts and seeds. This recommendation can be particularly healthful if these vegetable foods are substitutes for red meat, chicken, eggs, and dairy products.

■ Eat small amounts of avocados and include monounsaturated oils, such as olive, canola, and hazelnut, as a dressing on your vegetables and salads, or in your cooking.

■ Nut butters—peanut, sesame, and almond—should be used sparingly. Nut butters that have been hydrogenated or contain salt should be avoided by people with coronary heart disease and hypertension.

■ People with high blood pressure but healthy cholesterol levels may increase their intake of cold-water fish such as salmon, mackerel, and sardines.

■ Limit high-satiety vegetables to four servings daily and high-satiety fruits to three servings each day.

■ Do not overeat, no matter what your weight.

As I have demonstrated throughout this book, the Pritikin Program can be modified and adapted to virtually any situation or health condition. Use the basic program described in chapter 7 and adopt the changes recommended here to suit your particular needs and condition. Your individualized program can bring about rapid results and a dramatic transformation of your health.

References

Introduction

Foods difficult to give up are those with fat, sugar:

Kanarek RB, Ryu M, and Przypek J. "Preferences for Foods with Varying Levels of Salt and Fat Differ as a Function of Dietary Restraint and Exercise but not Menstrual Cycle." *Physiology and Behavior*, 1995 May, 57(5):821–6.

Lahteenmaki L and Tuorila H. "Three-Factor Eating Questionnaire and the Use and Liking of Sweet and Fat among Dieters." *Physiology and Behavior*, 1995 January, 57(1):81–8.

Rolls, B.J. "Carbohydrates, Fats, and Satiety." *American Journal of Clinical Nutrition*, 1995 April, 61(4 Suppl):960S–967S.

People suffering from same underlying illness: poisoning of the body by excess fat, calories, cholesterol:

Toshima H., Koga Y., and Blackburn H. (eds.). "Lessons for Science from the Seven Countries Study: a 35-year Collaborative Experience in Cardiovascular Disease Epidemiology." Tokyo: Springer-Verlag, 1994.

40%W, 20% M on diets:

Kuczmarski R.J., Flegal K.M., Campbell S.M., and Johnson C.L. "Increasing Prevalence of Overweight among U.S. Adults." *Journal of the American Medical Association*, 1994;272:205–211.

"Losing Weight. What Works. What Doesn't." *Consumer Reports*, 1993, June: 347–357.

NIH Technology Assessment Conference Panel. "Methods for Voluntary Weight Loss and Control." *Annals of Internal Medicine*, 1993; 119:764–770.

Obesity epidemic in West:

Seidell, J.C. "Obesity in Europe: Scaling an Epidemic." *International Journal of Obesity and Related Metabolic Disorders*, 1995 September, 19 Suppl 3:S1–4.

"Update: Prevalence of Overweight among Children, Adolescents, and Adults—United States, 1988–1994." *MMWR. Morbidity and Mortality Weekly Report*, 1997 March 7, 46(9):198–202.

Heart disease equals number one killer:

From the Centers for Disease Control and Prevention. "Trends in Ischemic Heart Disease Deaths—United States, 1990–1994." *JAMA,* 1997 April 9, 277(14):1109.

Verschuren W.M., Jacobs D.R., Bloemberg B.P., Kromhout D., Menotti A., Aravanis C., Blackburn H., Buzina R., Dontas A.S., and Fidanza F., et al. "Serum Total Cholesterol and Long-term Coronary Heart Disease Mortality in Different Cultures. Twenty-five-year Follow-up of the Seven Countries Study." *JAMA,* 1995 July 12, 274(2):131–6.

Eating fat helped forbears survive famine:

Eaton S.B. "Humans, Lipids and Evolution." *Lipids,* 1992 October, 27(10):814–20.

Eaton S.B., Eaton S.B. III, Konner M.J., and Shostak M. "An Evolutionary Perspective Enhances Understanding of Human Nutritional Requirements." *Journal of Nutrition,* 1996 June, 126(6):1732–40.

Flatt, J.P. "Use and Storage of Carbohydrate and Fat." *American Journal of Clinical Nutrition,* 1995 April, 61(4 Suppl):952S–959S.

Rosenbaum M., Leibel R.L., Hirsch J. "Obesity." [Medical Progress] *New England Journal of Medicine,* 1997; 337:396–402.

Fat calories can be stored efficiently and used during famines:

Dulloo A.G., Jacquet J., and Girardier L. "Poststarvation Hyperphagia and Body Fat Overshooting in Humans: A Role for Feedback Signals from Lean and Fat Tissues." *American Journal of Clinical Nutrition,* 1997 March, 65(3):717–23.

Fat has been limited in previous human experience:

Eaton S.B. "Humans, Lipids and Evolution." *Lipids,* 1992 October 27(10):814–20.

We had to develop instinct for fat because it conferred survival advantage:

Eaton S.B. "Humans, Lipids and Evolution." *Lipids,* 1992 October, 27(10):814–20.

No sense of deprivation in adopting Pritikin approach:

Klem M.L., Wing R.R., McGuire M.T., Seagle H.M., Hill J.O. "A Descriptive Study of Individuals Successful at Long-term Maintenance of Substantial Weight Loss." *American Journal of Clinical Nutrition* 1997; 66:239–246.

Shah M., McGovern P., French S., and Baxter J. "Comparison of a Low-Fat, Ad Libitum Complex-Carbohydrate diet with a Low-energy Diet in Moderately Obese Women." *American Journal of Clinical Nutrition,* 1994; 59:980–984.

Men are scavengers; they gorged on fat when they could find it, especially after starvation:

Dulloo A.G., Jacquet J., and Girardier L. "Poststarvation Hyperphagia and Body Fat Overshooting in Humans: A Role for feedback signals from lean and fat tissues." *American Journal of Clinical Nutrition,* 1997 March, 65(3):717–23.

Eaton S.B. "Humans, Lipids and Evolution." *Lipids,* 1992 October, 27(10):814–20.

Dieting is like famine; encourages gorging:

Brownell K.D. and Rodin J. "Medical, Metabolic, and Psychological Effects of Weight Cycling." *Archives of Internal Medicine,* 1994 June 27, 154(12):1325–30.

Dulloo A.G., Jacquet J., and Girardier L. "Poststarvation Hyperphagia and Body Fat Overshooting in Humans: A Role for Feedback Signals from Lean and Fat Tissues." *American Journal of Clinical Nutrition,* 1997 March, 65(3):717–23.

Laessle R.G., Platte P., Schweiger U., and Pirke K.M. "Biological and Psychological Correlates of Intermittent Dieting Behavior in Young Women. A Model for Bulimia Nervosa." *Physiology and Behavior,* 1996 July, 60(1):1–5.

Polivy J., Zeitlin S.B., Herman C.P., and Beal A.L. "Food Restriction and Binge Eating: A Study of Former Prisoners of War." *Journal of Abnormal Psychology,* 1994 May, 103(2):409–11. (UI: 94315183)

Chapter 1: The Fat Instinct Revealed

In weight loss, the first 10 lbs are the easiest:

Weintraub M., Sundaresan P.R., Nadan M., Schuster B., Balder A., Lasagna I., and Cox C. "Long-Term Weight Control Study I. (weeks 0 to 34)." *Clinical Pharmacology and Therapy* 1992; 51:586–594.

Extra wt. increases risk of heart disease, diabetes, high blood pressure, and breast and ovarian cancer:

Andersson S.O., Wolk A., Bergstrom R., Adami H.O., Engholm G., Englund A., and Nyren O. "Body Size and Prostate Cancer: a 20-Year Follow-up Study among 135,006 Swedish Construction Workers." *Journal of the National Cancer Institute,* 1997 March 5, 89(5):385–9.

Carey V.J., Walters E.E., Colditz G.A., Solomon C.G., Willett W.C., Rosner B.A., Speizer F.E., and Manson J.E. "Body Fat Distribution and Risk of Non-insulin-dependent Diabetes Mellitus in Women: The Nurses' Health Study." *American Journal of Epidemiology,* 1997 April 1, 145(7):614–9.

DiPietro L., Mossberg H.O., and Stunkard A.J. "A 40-Year History of Overweight Children in Stockholm: Life-Time Overweight, Morbidity, and Mortality." *International Journal of Obesity and Related Metabolic Disorders,* 1994 September, 18(9):585–90.

Lamon-Fava S., Wilson P.W., and Schaefer E.J. "Impact of Body Mass Index on Coronary Heart Disease Risk Factors in Men and Women. The Framingham Offspring Study." *Arteriosclerosis, Thrombosis, and Vascular Biology,* 1996 December, 16(12):1509–15.

Lee, I.M., Manson J.E., Hennekens C.H., and Paffenbarger R.S., Jr. "Body Weight and Mortality: A 27-year Follow-up of Middle-aged Men." [see comments]. *JAMA,* 1993 December 15, 270(23):2823–8.

Peters E.T., Seidell J.C., Menotti A., Arayanis C., Dontas A., Fidanza F., Karvonen M., Nedeljkovic S., Nissinen A., Buzina R., et al. "Changes in Body Weight in Relation to Mortality in 6,441 European Middle-Aged men: The Seven Countries Study." *International Journal of Obesity and Related Metabolic Disorders,* 1995 December.

Seidell J.C., Verschuren W.M., van Leer E.M., and Kromhout D. "Overweight, Underweight, and Mortality. A Prospective Study of 48,287 Men and Women." *Archives of Internal Medicine*, 1996 May 13, 156(9):958–63.

Trentham-Dietz A., Newcomb P.A., Storer B.E., Longnecker M.P., Baron J., Greenberg E.R., and Willett W.C. "Body Size and Risk of Breast Cancer." *American Journal of Epidemiology*, 1997; 145:1011–1019.

"Update: Prevalence of Overweight among Children, Adolescents, and Adults— United States, 1988–1994." *MMWR. Morbidity and Mortality Weekly Report*, 1997 March 7, 46(9):198–202.

People who are fat are less attractive:

Gortmaker S.L., Must A., Perrin J.M., Sobol A.M., and Dietz W.H. "Social and Economic Consequences of Overweight in Adolescence and Young Adulthood." *New England Journal of Medicine*, 1993; 329(14):1008–12.

Skipping breakfast is not a good way to lose weight:

McNutt S.W., Hu Y., Schreiber G.B., Crawford P.B., Obarzanek E., Mellin L. "A Longitudinal Study of the Dietary Practices of Black and White Girls 9 and 10 Years Old at Enrollment: The NHLBI Growth and Health Study." *Journal of Adolescent Health*, 1997 January, 20(1):27–37.

Dieting contributes to poor mood:

Laessle R.G., Platte P., Schweiger U., and Pirke K.M. "Biological and Psychological Correlates of Intermittent Dieting Behavior in Young Women: A model for Bulimia Nervosa." *Physiology and Behavior*, 1996 July, 60(1):1–5.

5% of wt. losers are so disciplined, they can keep it off for 5 years:

"Losing Weight. What works. What doesn't." *Consumer Reports*, 1993, June:347–357.

Different foods give different experiences of satiety:

Holt, S.H.A., Brand-Miller J.C., Petocz P., and Farmakalidis E. "A Satiety Index of Common Foods." *European Journal of Clinical Nutrition*, 1995; 49:675–690.

Pennington J.A.T. *Bowes & Church's Food Values of Portions Commonly Used.* 16th edition. Philadelphia: Lippincott, 1994.

Vegetables tend to be rich in fiber, but low in calories:

Saldanha L.G. "Fiber in the Diet of US Children: Results of National Surveys." *Pediatrics*, 1995 November, 96(5 Pt 2):994–7.

Ursin G., Ziegler R.G., Subar A.F., Graubard B.I., Haile R.W., and Hoover R. "Dietary Patterns Associated with a Low-fat Diet in the National Health Examination Follow-up Study: Identification of Potential Confounders for Epidemiologic Analyses." *American Journal of Epidemiology*, 1993 April 15, 137(8):916–27.

Fruit is also low in calories, although not as low as veggies:

Pennington J.A.T. *Bowes & Church's Food Values of Portions Commonly Used.* 16th edition. Philadelphia: Lippincott, 1994.

Early humans had to exercise more than we do:

Eaton S.B. and Konner M. "Paleolithic nutrition: A Consideration of its Nature and Current Implications." *New England Journal of Medicine,* 1985; 312:283–289.

Early humans had only primitive tools for hunting:

Huang W., Ciochon R., Gu Y., Larick R., Qiren F., Schwarcz H., Yonge C., de Vos J., and Rink W. "Early Homo and Associated Artefacts from Asia." [see comments] *Nature,* 1995 November 16, 378(6554):275–8.

Early humans did not get as much fat from animal foods as we do, pound for pound:

Eaton S.B. and Konner M. "Paleolithic nutrition: A Consideration of its Nature and Current Implications." *New England Journal of Medicine,* 1985; 312:283–289.
Eaton S.B., Konner M., and Shostak M. "Stone Agers in the Fast Lane: Chronic Degenerative Diseases in Evolutionary Perspective." *American Journal of Medicine,* 1988 April, 84(4):739–49.
Rosenbaum M., Leibel R.I., Hirsch J. "Obesity." [Medical Progress] *New England Journal of Medicine* 1997; 337:396–402.

Nature has programmed us, as adults, to conserve energy by preferring sedentariness:

Ibid.

Humans decrease metabolic rate in face of famine:

Leibel R.L., Rosenbaum M., and Hirsch J. "Changes in Energy Expenditure Resulting from Altered Body Weight." *The New England Journal of Medicine,* 1995; 332:621–628.

Calorie restriction produces many changes, including headaches, fatigue, weakness, anxiety, and craving for calorie dense foods:

Keys A., Brozek J., Henschel A., Mickelsen O., and Taylor H.L. *The Biology of Human Starvation.* Minneapolis: University of Minnesota Press, 1950.
Laessle R.G., Platte P., Schweiger U., and Pirke K.M. "Biological and Psychological Correlates of Intermittent Dieting Behavior in Young Women." A model for Bulimia Nervosa." *Physiology and Behavior,* 1996 July, 60(1):1–5.

Only in last 60 years have westerners managed to bring food supply under control and provide abundance of fat:

Trowell H. "Obesity in the Western World." *Plant Foods for Man,* 1975; 1:157–168.

Cancer kills more than ¹/₂ million Americans each year and affects 1 out of 3 Americans over a lifetime:

(Statistics obtained from the American Cancer Society WWW page 6/5/97 at: http://www.cancer.org/97facts.html.)

Cardiovascular disease affects more than 50 million and accounts for more than 40% of all deaths (over 900,000 deaths/year):

(Statistics obtained from the American Heart Association WWW page at: http://www.amhrt.org/1997/stats/CardDise.html.)

Diabetes affects more than 13 million Americans:

Geiss L.S., Herman W.H., Goldschmid M.G., DeStefano F., Eberhardt M.S., Ford E.S., German R.R., Newman J.M., Olson D.R., Sepe S.J., et al. "Surveillance for Diabetes Mellitus—United States, 1980–1989." *MMWR CDC Surveillance Summaries,* 1993 June 4, 42(2):1–20.

More than 50% of Americans are substantially over their medically desirable weight and nearly 33% are obese (> 120% of medically desirable body weight):

"Update: Prevalence of Overweight among Children, Adolescents, and Adults— United States, 1988–1994." *MMWR. Morbidity and Mortality Weekly Report,* 1997 March 7, 46(9):198–202.

Dietary fat is healthful in small doses but lethal in excess:

National Research Council. *Recommended Dietary Allowances.* Washington, D.C.: National Academy Press, 1989. "Lipids," pp. 44–51.

U.S. Department of Health and Human Services. *The Surgeon General's Report on Nutrition and Health.* DHHS (PHS) Publication No. 88-50210. Washington, D.C.: U.S. Government Printing Office, 1988.

Darwin, Charles, 1809–1882. *The Origin of Species.* London: J.M. Dent & Sons; New York: E.P. Dutton [1951].

Body requires only 20 minutes of sun each day to get enough vitamin D:

National Research Council. *Recommended Dietary Allowances.* Washington, D.C.: National Academy Press, 1989. "Fat-soluble vitamins," pp. 92–98.

Adopting a more plant-based diet tends to make nutrient levels go up:

Gorbach, S.L., Morrill-LaBrode, A., Woods, M.N., Dwyer, J.T., Selles, W.D., Henderson, M., Insull, W., Goldman, S., Thompson, D., Clifford, C., Sheppard, L. (1990). "Changes in Food Patterns During a Low-Fat Dietary Intervention in Women." *Journal of the American Dietetic Association,* 90, 802–809.

Ursin G., Ziegler R.G., Subar A.F., Graubard B.I., Haile R.W., Hoover R. "Dietary Patterns Associated with a Low-fat Diet in the National Health Examination Follow-up Study: Identification of Potential Confounders for Epidemiologic Analyses" [see comments]. *American Journal of Epidemiology,* 1993 April 15, 137(8):916–27.

Attenborough, David, 1926– *Life on Earth: A Natural History*. 1st American edition. Boston: Little, Brown, 1979.

Eaton S.B. and Konner M. "Paleolithic Nutrition: A Consideration of Its Nature and Current Implications." *New England Journal of Medicine*, 1985; 312:283–289.

Trowell H., Burkitt D., Heaton K., eds. *Dietary Fibre, Fibre-depleted Foods and Disease*. Foreword by Sir Richard Doll. London; Orlando: Academic Press, 1985.

Truswell, A. Stewart. *ABC of Nutrition*; with contributions from Brand J.C., Irving M., and Noah N.D. London: British Medical Association, 1986.

Herbivores have jaws that move sideways as well as vertically:

Cunningham, J.G., ed. *Textbook of Veterinary Physiology*. Philadelphia: Saunders, 1992.

Human saliva is different from that of carnivores; carnivores' saliva is acidic. Human saliva is alkaline and contains dietary enzyme, amylase:

Ibid.
Fox, Stuart Ira. *Human Physiology*. 4th edition. Dubuque, Iowa: W.C. Brown, 1993.

Human digestive tract is long and meandering, like those of herbivores, unlike carnivores:

Cunningham J.G., ed. *Textbook of Veterinary Physiology*. Philadelphia: Saunders, 1992.
Fox, Stuart Ira. *Human Physiology*. 4th edition. Dubuque, Iowa: W.C. Brown, 1993.

Humans can store 5–7 year supply of vitamin B12:

National Research Council. *Diet and Health. Implications for Reducing Chronic Disease Risk*. Washington, D.C.: National Academy Press, 1989. "Water soluble vitamins, pp. 158–164.

Humans can generate all the cholesterol they need:

National Research Council. *Diet and Health. Implications for Reducing Chronic Disease Risk*. Washington, D.C.: National Academy Press, 1989. "Lipids," pp. 44–51.

Campbell has determined that serum cholesterol is best marker in Chinese person of serious illness:

Campbell T.C. and Junshi C. "Diet and Chronic Degenerative Diseases: Perspectives from China." *American Journal of Clinical Nutrition*, 1994 May, 59(5 Suppl): 1153S–1161S.

Paleolithic ancestors ate at least 3x more plant foods than we do today:

Eaton S.B., Konner M. "Paleolithic Nutrition: A Consideration of Its Nature and Current Implications." *New England Journal of Medicine*, 1985; 312:283–289.

Gaster, T.H. The New Golden Bough (originally authored by Frazer):

Frazer, James George, Sir, 1854–1941. *The New Golden Bough: A New Abridgment of the Classic Work.* Edited, and with notes and foreword by Theodor H. Gaster. New York: Criterion Books [1959].

Ravussin E., Valencia M.E., Esparza J., Bennett P.H., and Schulz L.O. "Effects of a Traditional Lifestyle on Obesity in Pima Indians." *Diabetes Care* 1994; 17; 1067–1074.

When Japanese immigrants came to U.S., they began to suffer same chronic diseases as other Americans:

Brown J., Bourke G.J., Gearty G.F., and Finnegan A., et al. "Nutritional and Epidemiologic Factors Related to Heart Disease." *World Reviews in Nutrition and Diet.* 1970; 12:1–42.
Chen J., Campbell T.C., Peto R.J., and Li J. *Diet, Life-style and Mortality in China: A Study of the Characteristics of 65 Chinese Counties.* Oxford: Oxford University Press; Ithaca, NY: Cornell University Press; People's Republic of China: People's Medical Pub. House, 1990.

Rural Chinese eat more calories than U.S. residents do:

Ibid.
Lee M.M., Wu-Williams A., Whittemore A.S., and Zheng S., et al. "Comparison of Dietary Habits, Physical Activity and Body Size among Chinese in North America and China." *International Journal of Epidemiology* 1994; 23:984–990.

Obesity has traditionally been rare in China:

Chen J., Campbell T.C., Peto R.J., and Li J. *Diet, Life-style and Mortality in China: A Study of the Characteristics of 65 Chinese Counties.* Oxford: Oxford University Press; Ithaca, NY: Cornell University Press; People's Republic of China: People's Medical Pub. House, 1990.
Lee M.M., Wu-Williams A., Whittemore A.S., and Zheng S., et al. "Comparison of Dietary Habits, Physical Activity and Body Size among Chinese in North America and China." *International Journal of Epidemiology,* 1994; 23:984–990.

They eat 60% less fat and a third less protein. 93% of protein comes from plant sources, as opposed to U.S. 30%:

Chen J., Campbell T.C., Peto R.J., and Li J. *Diet, Life-style and Mortality in China: A Study of the Characteristics of 65 Chinese Counties.* Oxford: Oxford University Press; Ithaca, NY: Cornell University Press; People's Republic of China: People's Medical Pub. House, 1990.

Pritikin accomplishments:

Decrease cholesterol and triglycerides:

Barnard R.J. "Effects of Life-style Modification on Serum Lipids." *Archives of Internal Medicine,* 1991; 151:1389–1394.

Decrease high blood pressure:

Barnard R.J., Jung T., and Inkeles S.B. "Diet and Exercise in the Treatment of NIDDM: The Need for Early Emphasis." *Diabetes Care,* 1994 December, 17(12):1469–72.

Barnard R.J., Ugianskis E.J., Martin D.A., and Inkeles S.B. "Role of Diet and Exercise in the Management of Hyperinsulinemia and Associated Atherosclerotic Risk Factors." *American Journal of Cardiology,* 1992 February 15, 69(5):440–4.

Decrease angina and number of candidates for coronary bypass surgery:

Hall J.A. and Barnard R.J. "The effects of an Intensive 26-Day Program of Diet and Exercise on Patients with Peripheral Vascular Disease." *Journal of Cardiac Rehabilitation,* 1982; 2:569–574.

Improve symptoms of diabetes:

Barnard R.J., Jung T., and Inkeles S.B. "Diet and Exercise in the Treatment of NIDDM." *Diabetes Care,* 1994; 17:1469–1472.

Barnard R.J., Massey M.R., Cherny S., O'Brien L.T., and Pritikin N. "Long-Term Use of a High-Complex-Carbohydrate, High-fiber, Low-fat Diet and Exercise in the Treatment of NIDDM Patients." *Diabetes Care,* 1983 May–June, 6(3):268–73.

Barnard R.J., Ugianskis E.J., Martin D.A., and Inkeles S.B. "Role of Diet and Exercise in the Management of Hyperinsulinemia and Associated Atherosclerotic Risk Factors." *American Journal of Cardiology,* 1992 February 15, 69(5):440–4.

Ibid.

Reduce risks of breast and colon cancer:

Bagga D., Ashley J.M., Geffrey S., Wang H-J., Barnard J., Elashoff R., and Heber D. "Modulation of Serum and Breast Ductal Fluid Lipids by a Very Low-fat, High-fiber Diet in Premenopausal Women." *Journal of the National Cancer Institute,* 1994; 86:1419–1421.

Bagga D., Ashley J.M., Geffrey S.P., and Wang H.J., et al. "Effects of a Very Low-Fat, High-Fiber Diet on Serum Hormones and Menstrual Function-Implications for Breast Cancer Prevention." *Cancer,* 1995; 76:2491–2496.

Reddy B.S., Engle A., Simi B., O'Brien L.T., Barnard R.J., Pritikin N., and Wynder E.L. "Effect of Low-fat, High-carbohydrate, High-fiber Diet on Fecal Bile Acids and Neutral Sterols." *Preventive Medicine,* 1988; 17:432–439.

Native Hawaiians are almost uniformly obese and live shorter lives:

Braun K.L., Yang H., Onaka A.T., and Horiuchi B.Y. "Life and Death in Hawaii: Ethnic Variations in Life Expectancy and Mortality, 1980 and 1990." *Hawaii Medical Journal,* 1996 December, 55(12):278–83, 302.

Historical accounts show that native Hawaiians were originally slim:

Shintani T.T., Hughes C.K., Beckham S., and O'Connor H.K. "Obesity and Cardiovascular Risk Intervention Through the Ad Libitum Feeding of Traditional Hawaiian Diet." *American Journal of Clinical Nutrition,* 1991; 53:1647S–1651S.

Holt S.H.A., Brand-Miller J.C., Petocz P., and Farmakalidis E. "A Satiety Index of Common Foods." *European Journal of Clinical Nutrition*, 1995; 49:675–690.

Chapter 3: Why Dieting Fails in America

Fifty million Americans are dieting right now:

NIH Technology Assessment Conference Panel. "Methods for Voluntary Weight Loss and Control." *Annals of Internal Medicine*, 1993; 119:764–770.

The range of major strategies for achieving weight loss:

NIH Technology Assessment Conference Panel. "Methods for Voluntary Weigh Loss and Control." *Annals of Internal Medicine*, 1993; 119:764–770.

Symptoms reflecting the famine response:

Keys A., Brozek J., Henschel A., Mickelsen O., and Taylor HL. *The Biology of Human Starvation.* Minneapolis: University of Minnesota Press, 1950.

People lack energy, show irritability, are more prone to depression when dieting:

Ibid.

Body slows down metabolism in face of famine, to conserve calories:

Leibel R.L., Rosenbaum M., and Hirsch J. "Changes in Energy Expenditure Resulting from Altered Body Weight." *The New England Journal of Medicine*, 1995 332:621–628.

Body is capable of less work when glycogen stores are kept half empty:

Immediately after end of bout of dieting, body is prone to regain weight faster with baseline level of calorie intake than was case before dieting:

In immediate post-famine mode, body tends to gorge:

Keys A., Brozek J., Henschel A., Mickelsen O., and Taylor H.L. *The Biology of Human Starvation.* Minneapolis: University of Minnesota Press, 1950.

Lissner, L., Levitsky, D.A., Strupp, B.J., Kalkwarf, H.J., and Roe, D.A. "Dietary Fat and the Regulation of energy Intake in Human Subjects." American Journal of Clinical Nutrition, 1987; 46:886–892.

Kendall A., Levitsky D.A., Strupp B.J., and Lissner L. "Weight Loss on a Low-fat Diet: Consequence of the Imprecision of the Control of Food Intake in Humans." *American Journal of Clinical Nutrition*, 1991; 53:1124–1129.

Diamond J. Natural History 1992 February; 2–6.

Holt S.H.A., Brand-Miller J.C., Petocz P., and Farmakalidis E. "A Satiety Index of Common Foods." *European Journal of Clinical Nutrition*, 1995; 49:675–690.

Kenny J. *American J. Clinical Nutrition*, 1992; 2(1): 81–93.

Lovejoy J., et al. *American Journal of Clinical Nutrition*, 1992; 55:1174–1179.

Ravussin E. *Diabetes Care*, 1994; 17(9):1067–1074.

Ordinarily, the brain's only fuel is glucose:

Bonadonna R.C. and DeFronzo R.A. Chapter 40. "Glucose Metabolism in Obesity and Type II Diabetes." In P. Bjorntorp, B.N. Brodoff, eds., *Obesity*. Philadelphia: Lippincott, 1994. pp. 474–501.

Body can convert triglycerides to ketones, to fuel brain on emergency basis when brain glucose levels are too low:

Owen O.E., et al. "Brain Metabolism during Fasting." *Journal of Clinical Investigation*, 1967; 46:1589–1595.

Symptoms and problems associated with ketosis:

Van Itallie T.B. "Diets for Weight Reduction: Mechanisms of Action and Physiological Effects." In Bray G., ed. *Obesity: Comparative Methods of Weight Control*. London: John Libbey, 1980.

Wing R.R., Vazquez J.A., and Ryan C.M. "Cognitive Effects of Ketogenic Weight-reducing Diets." *International Journal of Obesity and Related Metabolic Disorders*, 1995 November, 19(11):811–6.

AMA Encyclopedia of Medicine:

Clayman C.B., medical ed. *The American Medical Association Encyclopedia of Medicine*. New York, NY: Random House, 1989.

Eades M.R. and Eades M.D. Protein Power. *Bantam. 1996:*

Eades, M.D. and M.R. *Protein Power: The Metabolic Breakthrough*. New York: Bantam Books, 1996.

Abundant evidence shows that high-protein diets contribute to variety of conditions:

Beltz S.D. and Doering P.L. "Efficacy of Nutritional Supplements used by Athletes." *Clinical Pharmacy*, 1993 December, 12(12):900–8.

Feskanich D., Willett W.C., Stampfer M.J., and Colditz G.A. "Protein Consumption and Bone Fractures in Women." *American Journal of Epidemiology*, 1996 March 1, 143(5):472–9.

Toniolo P., Riboli E., Shore R.E., and Pasternack B.S. "Consumption of Meat, Animal Products, Protein, and Fat and Risk of Breast Cancer: A Prospective Cohort Study in New York." [see comments] *Epidemiology*, 1994 July, 5(4):391–7.

ACS, AHA, USDA, NRC guidelines:

American Cancer Society. "Guidelines on Diet, Nutrition, and Cancer Prevention: Reducing the Risk of Cancer with Healthy Food Choices and Physical Activity." *CA: Cancer Journal for Clinicians*, 1996; 46:325–341.

Krauss R.M., Deckelbaum R.J., Ernst N., Fisher E., Howard B.V., and Knopp R.H., et al. "Dietary Guidelines for Healthy American Adults." *Circulation*, 1996; 94:1795–1800.

National Research Council. *Diet and Health: Implications for Reducing Chronic Disease Risk.* Washington, D.C.: National Academy Press, 1989.

U.S. Department of Agriculture & U.S. Department of Health and Human Services. *Dietary Guidelines for Americans.* Fourth Edition. Home and Garden Bulletin No. 232. Washington, D.C.: U.S. Government Printing Office, 1995.

Hunger for carbohydrates is great when body is in ketosis, as during starvation:

Keys A., Brozek J., Henschel A., Mickelsen O., and Taylor H.L. *The Biology of Human Starvation.* Minneapolis: University of Minnesota Press, 1950.

Calorie restriction leads to weight regain 95% of the time:

"Losing Weight. What works. What doesn't." *Consumer Reports,* 1993, June issue: 347–357.

Exercise is associated with preserving lean body tissue during weight loss, relative to calorie restriction, and relative to ketogenic diets:

Skender M.L., Goodrick G.K., Del Junco D.J., Reeves R.S., Darnell L., Gotto A.M., and Foreyt J.P. "Comparison of Two-Year Weight Loss Trends in Behavioral Treatments of Obesity: Diet, Exercise, and Combination Interventions." *Journal of the American Dietetic Association,* 1996 April, 96(4):342–6.

Vazquez J.A. and Adibi S.A. "Protein Sparing during Treatment of Obesity: Ketogenic versus Nonketogenic Very Low Calorie Diet." *Metabolism: Clinical and Experimental,* 1992 April, 41(4):406–14.

Zachwieja J.J. "Exercise as Treatment for Obesity." *Endocrinology and Metabolism Clinics of North America,* 1996 December.

Pleasure Revenge, *by Faith Popcorn:*

Hochstein, Mort. "Pleasure Revenge" or Hard Work Well Done?" *Nation's Restaurant News,* v.28, n.20 (May 16, 1994):53.

Chapter 4. Weight Loss Without Hunger

Plant foods are basis of effective weight control:

Campbell T.C. and Junshi C. "Diet and Chronic Degenerative Diseases: Perspectives from China." *American Journal of Clinical Nutrition,* 1994 May, 59(5 Suppl): 1153S–1161S.

Jenkins D.J. "Optimal Diet for Reducing the Risk of Arteriosclerosis." *Canadian Journal of Cardiology,* 1995 October, 11 Suppl G:118G–122G.

"Science is showing that micronutrients, phytonutrients and other antioxidants are important for preventing mutations, cancers, heart disease, and boosting immune system:

Ames B.N., Gold L.S., and Willett W.C. "The Causes and Prevention of Cancer." *Proceedings of the National Academy of Sciences of the United States of America,* 1995 June 6, 92(12):5258–65.

Alpha-Tocopherol, Beta Carotene Cancer Prevention Study Group. "The Effect of

Vitamin E and Beta Carotene on the Incidence of Lung Cancer and Other Cancers in Male Smokers." *New England Journal of Medicine*, 1994; 330:1029–1035.

Harbige L.S. "Nutrition and Immunity with Emphasis on Infection and Autoimmune Disease." *Nutrition and Health*, 1996, 10(4):285–312.

Hennekens C.H. "Antioxidant Vitamins and Cardiovascular Disease: Current Perspectives and Future Directions." Editorial. *European Heart Journal*, 1997 February 18(2):177–9.

Omenn G.S., Goodman G.E., Thornquist M.D., Balmes J., Cullen M.R., Glass A., Keogh J.P., Meyskens F.L., Valanis B., and Williams J.H., et al. "Effects of a Combination of Beta Carotene and Vitamin A on Lung Cancer and Cardiovascular Disease." *New England Journal of Medicine*, 1996; 334:1150–5.

Plants are good sources, animals are poor sources of many antioxidants and phytonutrients:

Ames B.N., Gold L.S., and Willett W.C. "The Causes and Prevention of Cancer." *Proceedings of the National Academy of Sciences of the United States of America*, 1995 June 6, 92(12):5258–65.

Campbell T.C. and Junshi C. "Diet and Chronic Degenerative Diseases: Perspectives from China." *American Journal of Clinical Nutrition*, 1994 May, 59(5 Suppl): 1153S–1161S.

Jenkins D.J. "Optimal Diet for Reducing the Risk of Arteriosclerosis." *Canadian Journal of Cardiology*, 1995 October, 11 (Suppl G):118G–122G.

Chapter 5: Carbohydrates: The Real Story

Not all carbohydrates are created equal; processed carbohydrates, which typically have less fiber or water than minimally processed plant foods, produce higher levels of blood glucose and insulin when consumed in quantity:

Jenkins D. "Wholemeal Versus Wholegrain Breads: Proportion of Whole or Cracked Grain and the Glycemic Index." *British Medical Journal* 1988; 297:958.

Jenkins D. "Effect of Processing on Digestibility and the Blood Glucose Response: A Study of Lentils." *American Journal of Clinical Nutrition*, 1982; 36:1093–

Haber G. "Depletion and Disruption of Dietary Fiber. Effects on Satiety, Plasma-Glucose, and Serum-Insulin." *Lancet*, 1977; 2:679.

O'Dea K. "Physical Factors Influencing Postprandial Glucose and Insulin Responses to Starch." *American Journal of Clinical Nutrition*, 1980; 33:760.

O'Dea K. "The Rate of Starch Hydrolysis In Vitro as a Predictor of Metabolic Responses to Complex Carbohydrates In Vivo." *American Journal of Clinical Nutrition*, 1981; 34:1991.

Eating fat and sugar together produces more deleterious changes in blood values:

Suzuki M. "Simultaneous Ingestion of Fat and Sucrose may Contribute to Development of Obesity: A Larger Body Fat Accumulation as Compared with Their Separate Ingestion." *Federation Proceedings*, 1986; 45:481.

Slowing down absorption via fiber, "resistant" starch or by distributing carbohydrate calories over more frequent, smaller meals produces better blood values:

Jenkins D.J., Jenkins A.L., Wolever T.M., Vuksan V., Rao A.V., Thompson L.U., and Josse R.G. "Low Glycemic Index: Lente Carbohydrates and Physiological Effects of Altered Food Frequency." *American Journal of Clinical Nutrition*, 1994, 59:706S–709S.

The body tries to protect itself from enduringly high levels of blood glucose by producing more insulin:

Barnard R.J., Youngren J.F., and Martin D.A. "Diet, Not Aging, Causes Skeletal Muscle Insulin Resistance." *Gerontology*, 1995, 41(4):205–11.

Eckel R. "Insulin Resistance: An Adaptation for Weight Maintenance. *Lancet*, 1990; 340:1452.

The liver's capacity to store glycogen is significantly less than that of the muscles:

Coyle E.F. "Substrate Utilization during Exercise in Active People." *American Journal of Clinical Nutrition*, 1995 April, 61(4 Suppl):968S–979S.

Cunningham J.G., ed. *Textbook of Veterinary Physiology*. Philadelphia: Saunders, 1992.

The average woman's muscles can store 1000 kcal; the average man's muscles can store 1500 kcal of glycogen:

Cunningham J.G., ed. *Textbook of Veterinary Physiology*. Philadelphia: Saunders, 1992.

Vigorous, sustained exercise tends to deplete the muscles of glycogen:

Coyle E.F. "Substrate Utilization during Exercise in Active People." *American Journal of Clinical Nutrition*, 1995 April, 61(4 Suppl):968S–979S.

Excess sugar is rarely converted to fat:

Acheson K.J., Schutz Y., Bessard T., Anantharaman K., Flatt J.P., and Jequier E. "Glycogen Storage Capacity and De Novo Lipogenesis during Massive Carbohydrate Overfeeding in Man." *American Journal of Clinical Nutrition*, 1988 August, 48(2):240–7.

Jebb S.A., Prentice A.M., Goldberg G.R., Murgatroyd P.R., Black A.E., and Coward W.A. "Changes in Macronutrient Balance during Over- and Underfeeding Assessed by 12-d Continuous Whole-body Calorimetry. *American Journal of Clinical Nutrition*, 1996 September, 64(3):259–66.

Stored fat is eight times lighter, calorie for calorie, then stored glycogen or protein:

Flatt J.P. "McCollum Award Lecture, 1995: Diet, Lifestyle, and Weight Maintenance. *American Journal of Clinical Nutrition*, 1995 October, 62(4):820–36.

When liver glycogen stores are full, appetite is suppressed for hours:

Raben A., Holst J.J., Christensen N.J., and Astrup A. "Determinants of Postprandial Appetite Sensations: Macronutrient Intake and Glucose Metabolism." *Inter-*

national Journal of Obesity and Related Metabolic Disorders, 1996 February 20(2):161–9.

Average American is probably burning about 50-50% carbohydrate/fat mix right now, as we speak. . . .:

McArdle W.D., Katch F.I., and Katch V.L. *Essentials of Exercise Physiology*. Philadelphia: Lea & Febiger, 1994.

Cooked oatmeal has greater satiety value than low-fiber dry cereal:

Turconi G., Gazzano R., Caramella R., Porrini M., Crovetti R., and Lanzola E. "The Effects of High Intakes of Fibre Ingested at Breakfast on Satiety." *European Journal of Clinical Nutrition*, 1995 October, 49 Supplement 3:S281–5.

Pasta is a salient exception, where processing has produced slower-to-absorb carbohydrate:

Jenkins D. "Effect of Processing on Digestibility and the Blood Glucose Response: A Study of Lentils." *American Journal of Clinical Nutrition*, 1982; 36:1093.

Eating a diet of vegetables, beans, fruit and minimally processed grains will keep calories and insulin levels low:

Jenkins D.J. Optimal Diet for Reducing the Risk of Arteriosclerosis. *Canadian Journal of Cardiology*, 1995 October, 11 Supplement G:118G–122G.

Sugar is almost as bad as fat for increasing intake of total calories and conducing to obesity:

Rolls B.J. "Carbohydrates, Fats, and Satiety." *American Journal of Clinical Nutrition*, 1995 April, 61 Supplement 4: 960S–967S.

Geiselman P.J. "Sugar-induced Hyperphagia: Is Hyperinsulinemia, Hypoglycemia, or Any Other Factor a "Necessary" Condition?" *Appetite*, 1988, 11 Supplement 1:26–34.

When diabetics start taking insulin, their hunger increases and they experience weight gain:

"Effect of Intensive Diabetes Management on Macrovascular Events and Risk Factors in the Diabetes Control and Complications Trial." *American Journal of Cardiology*, 1995 May 1, 75(14):894–903.

Hunger and the fat instinct defeat 95% of dieters in the long run:

"Losing Weight. What Works. What Doesn't." *Consumer Reports*, 1993, June: 347–357.

Dietary restraint; many Americans are "restrained eaters.":

Marcus M.D., Wing R.R., and Lamparski D.M. "Binge Eating and Dietary Restraint in Obese Patients." *Addictive Behaviors*, 1985, 10(2):163–8.

Over time, with increased exercise and continued exposure to lower-fat, lower-sodium foods you can come to prefer eating minimally processed carbohydrates:

Beauchamp G.K., Bertino M., and Engelman K. "Modification of Salt Taste. *Annals of Internal Medicine,* 1983; 98 (Part 2):763–769.

Epstein L.H., Valoski A., Wing R.R., Perkins K.A., Fernstrom M., Marks B., and McCurley J. "Perception of Eating and Exercise in Children as a Function of Child and Parent Weight Status." *Appetite,* 1989 April, 12(2):105–18.

Mattes R.D. "Fat Preference and Adherence to a Reduced-fat Diet." *American Journal of Clinical Nutrition,* 1993, 57(3):373–81.

Chapter 6: The Behaviors that Outsmart the Fat Instinct

Known for decades that diet that promotes optimal well-being is composed chiefly of fresh veggies, beans, fruit, whole grains, low-fat animal foods, and non-fat milk:

Campbell T.C. and Junshi C. Diet and Chronic Degenerative Diseases: Perspectives from China." *American Journal of Clinical Nutrition,* 1994 May, 59(5 Suppl): 1153S–1161S.

Eaton S.B. and Konner M. Paleolithic nutrition. "A Consideration of Its Nature and Current Implications." *New England Journal of Medicine,* 1985; 312:283–289.

Jenkins D.J. "Optimal Diet for Reducing the Risk of Arteriosclerosis." *Canadian Journal of Cardiology,* 1995 October, 11 Suppl G:118G–122G.

[It] provides max, nutrition, including the micronutrients that protect against major diseases:

Campbell T.C. and Junshi C. "Diet and Chronic Degenerative Diseases: Perspectives from China." *American Journal of Clinical Nutrition,* 1994 May, 59(5 Suppl): 1153S–1161S.

Pattern of our ancestors, relying upon plant sources, with occasional supplementation by animal foods:

Eaton S.B. and Konner M. "Paleolithic Nutrition: A Consideration of Its Nature and Current Implications." *New England Journal of Medicine,* 1985; 312:283–289.

Animals they did eat were low in fat because such animals were wild . . . different from farm-raised animals:

Eaton S.B. and Konner M. "Paleolithic Nutrition: A Consideration of Its Nature and Current Implications." *New England Journal of Medicine,* 1985; 312:283–289.

We store about 1500 kcal of energy from carb's versus 100,000–300,000 kcal in our fat stores . . .:

Flatt J.P. "Use and Storage of Carbohydrate and Fat." *American Journal of Clinical Nutrition,* 1995 April, 61(4 Suppl):952S–959S.

Those who exercise stand best chance of keeping excess weight off:

Grilo C.M., Brownell K.D., and Stunkard A.J. "The Metabolic and Psychological Importance of Exercise in Weight Control." In AJ Stunkard, TA Wadden eds., *Obesity: Theory and Therapy.* Second Edition New York: Raven Press, 1993, pp. 253–273.

Rosenbaum M., Leibel R.L., Hirsch J. "Obesity." [Medical Progress] *New England Journal of Medicine* 1997; 337:396–402.

Klem M.L., Wing R.R., McGuire M.T., Seagle H.M., and Hill J.O. "A Descriptive Study of Individuals Successful at Long-term Maintenance of Substantial Weight Loss." *American Journal of Clinical Nutrition* 1997; 66:239–246.

Those who rely on diet alone are most likely to fail in less than one year:

"Losing Weight. What Works. What Doesn't." *Consumer Reports,* 1993, June issue:347–357.

Gerardo-Gettens T., Miller G.D., Horwitz B.A., McDonald R.B., Brownell K.D., Greenwood M.R., Rodin J., and Stern J.S. "Exercise Decreases Fat Selection in Female Rats during Weight Cycling." *American Journal of Physiology,* 1991; 260:R518–24.

Simoes E.J., Byers T., Coates R.J., Serdula M.K., Mokdad A.H., and Heath G.W. "The Association Between Leisure-Time Physical Activity and Dietary Fat in American Adults." [see comments] *American Journal of Public Health,* 1995 February, 85(2):240–4.

Williams P.T. "High-Density Lipoprotein Cholesterol and Other Risk Factors for Coronary Heart Disease in Female Runners." [see comments]. *New England Journal of Medicine,* 1996 May 16, 334(20):1298–303.

Wood, P.D., Terry, R.B., and Haskell, W.L. "Metabolism of Substrates: diet, Lipoprotein Metabolism, and Exercise." *Federation Proceedings,* 1985; 44:358–363.

Eaton C.B., Reynes J., Assaf A.R., Feldman H., Lasater T., and Carleton R.A. "Predicting Physical Activity Change in Men and Women in Two New England Communities." *American Journal of Preventive Medicine,* 1993; 9:209–219.

Flatt J.P. "McCollum Award Lecture, 1995: Diet, Lifestyle, and Weight Maintenance." *American Journal of Clinical Nutrition,* 1995; 62:820–836.

Gerardo-Gettens T., Miller G.D., Horwitz B.A., McDonald R.G., Brownell K.D., Greenwood M.R.C., Rodin J., and Stern J.S. "Exercise Decreases Fat Selection in Female Rats during Weight Cycling." *American Journal Physiology,* 1991; 29:R518–R524.

Schaefer E.J., Lichtenstein A.H., Lamon-Fava S., McNamara J.R., Schaefer M.M., Rasmussen H., and Ordovas J.M. "Body Weight and Low-density Lipoprotein Cholesterol Changes after Consumption of a Low-fat Ad Libitum Diet." [see comments]. *Jama,* 1995 November 8, 274(18):1450–5.

Suddenly more carbs produces higher triglycerides:

Lichtenstein A.H., Ausman L.M., Carrasco W., Jenner J.L., Ordovas J.M., and Schaefer E.J. "Short-Term Consumption of a Low-fat Diet Beneficially Affects Plasma Lipid Concentrations Only When Accompanied by Weight loss. Hypercholesterolemia, Low-fat Diet, and Plasma Lipids." *Arteriosclerosis and Thrombosis,* 1994 November, 14(11):1751–60.

Higher triglycerides are associated with lower HDL's:

Tenkanen L., Pietila K., Manninen V., and Manttari M. "The triglyceride Issue Revisited. Findings from the Helsinki Heart Study." *Archives of Internal Medicine* 1994; 154:2714–2720.

U.S. Department of Agriculture & U.S. Department of Health and Human Services. *Dietary Guidelines for Americans.* Fourth Edition. Home and Garden Bulletin No. 232. Washington D.C.: U.S. Government Printing Office, 1995.

Most Americans are sedentary:

"State-specific Changes in Physical Inactivity among Persons Aged ≧ 65 Years— United States, 1987–1992." *MMWR. Morbidity and Mortality Weekly Report,* 1995 September 15, 44(36):663, 669, 672–3.

Calorie dense carbs plus fat can produce wt. gain despite exercise:

Lissner, L., Levitsky, D.A., Strupp, B.J., Kalkwarf, H.J., and Roe, D.A. "Dietary Fat and the Regulation of Energy Intake in Human Subjects." *American Journal of Clinical Nutrition,* 1987, 46:886–892.

Tremblay A., Almeras N., Boer J., Kranenbarg E.K., and Despres J-P. "Diet Composition and Postexercise Energy Balance." *American Journal of Clinical Nutrition,* 1994; 59:975–979.

Keep your insulin levels low, to permit high level of fat burning:

McArdle W.D., Katch F.I., Katch V.L. *Essentials of Exercise Physiology.* Philadelphia: Lea & Febiger, 1994.

Ancestors ate 12 servings a day:

Eaton S.B. and Konner M. "Paleolithic Nutrition. A Consideration of Its Nature and Current Implications." *New England Journal of Medicine,* 1985; 312:283–289.

Many Americans skip meals:

Lee C.J., Templeton S., and Wang C. "Meal Skipping Patterns and Nutrient Intakes of Rural Southern Elderly." *Journal of Nutrition for the Elderly,* 1996, 15(2):1–14.

McNutt S.W., Hu Y., Schreiber G.B., Crawford P.B., Obarzanek E., and Mellin L. "A Longitudinal Study of the Dietary Practices of Black and White Girls 9 and 10 Year Olds at Enrollment: The NHLBI Growth and Health Study." *Journal of Adolescent Health,* 1997 January, 20(1):27–37.

Americans' most popular lunch-time beverage is now a soft drink:

Jenkins D.J.A., Wolever, T.M.S., Vuksan V., Brighenti F., Cunnane S.C., Rao, A.V., Jenkins A.L., Buckley G., Patten R., Singer W., Corey P., and Josse R.G. "Nibbling versus Gorging: Metabolic Advantages of Increased Meal Frequency." *New England Journal of Medicine,* 1989; 321:929–934.

National Research Council. *Diet and Health: Implications for Reducing Chronic Disease Risk.* Washington, D.C.: National Academy Press, 1989.

Meal frequency may contribute to wt. loss, w/o going hungry:

Jenkins D.J., Jenkins A.L., Wolever T.M., Vuksan V., Rao A.V., Thompson L.U., and Josse R.G. "Low Glycemic Index: Lente Carbohydrates and Physiological Effects of Altered Food Frequency." *American Journal of Clinical Nutrition,* 1994 March, 59(3 Suppl):706S–709S.

Mattes R.D. "Fat Preference and Adherence to a Reduced-Fat Diet." *American Journal of Clinical Nutrition,* 1993; 57:373–381.

Ibid.

MRFIT study of consistency:

Combining exercise and diet is more effective for weight loss than either alone:

Patterson R.E., Haines P.S., and Popkin B.M. "Health Lifestyle Patterns of U.S. Adults." *Preventive Medicine,* 1994; 23:453–460.

Chapter 7: The Pritikin Program for Outsmarting the Fat Instinct

Immune systems get stronger:

Ames B.N., Gold L.S., and Willett W.C. "The Causes and Prevention of Cancer." *Proceedings of the National Academy of Sciences of the United States of America,* 1995 June 6, 92(12):5258–65.

Harbige L.S. "Nutrition and Immunity with Emphasis on Infection and Autoimmune Disease." *Nutrition and Health,* 1996, 10(4):285–312.

Consistency is the fastest and most efficient way to change your palate:

Mattes R.D. "Fat Preference and Adherence to a Reduced-Fat Diet." *American Journal of Clinical Nutrition,* 1993; 57:373–381.

For high-fat eaters who stick to low-fat diet consistently end up enjoying their low-fat foods:

Urban N., White E., Anderson G.L., Curry S., and Kristal A.R. "Correlates of Maintenance of a Low-fat Diet among Women in the Women's Health Trial." *Preventive Medicine,* 1992; 21:279–291.

Exercise increases craving for carbs and helps to lower body weight:

Wood P.D., Terry R.B., and Haskell W.L. "Metabolism of Substrates: Diet, Lipoprotein Metabolism, and Exercise." *Federation Proceedings,* 1985; 44:358–363.

Choose water-bearing, fiber-bearing carbs to help you lose weight:

Jenkins D.J., Jenkins A.L., Wolever T.M., Vuksan V., Rao A.V., Thompson L.U., and Josse R.G. "Low Glycemic Index: Lente Carbohydrates and Physiological Effects of Altered Food Frequency." *American Journal of Clinical Nutrition,* 1994; 59:706S–709S.

Eat less fat; it will promote health and weight loss:

Gorbach S.L., Morrill-LaBrode A., Woods M.N., Dwyer J.T., Selles W.D., Henderson M., Insull W., Goldman S., Thompson D., Clifford C., and Sheppard L. "Changes in Food Patterns during a Low-fat Dietary Intervention in Women." *Journal of the American Dietetic Association*, 1990; 90:802–809.

Haskell W.L., Alderman E.L., Fair J.M., Maron D.J., Mackey S.F., Superko H.R., Williams P.T., Johnstone I.M., Champagn M.A., Krauss R.M., and Farquhar J.W. "The Effects of Intensive Multiple Risk Factor Reduction on Coronary Atherosclerosis and Clinical Cardiac events in Men and Women with Coronary Artery Disease: The Stanford Coronary Risk Intervention Project (SCRIP)." *Circulation*, 1994; 89:975–990.

Eat frequently to keep burning fat and to prevent out-of-control hunger:

Jenkins D.J., Jenkins A.L., Wolever T.M., Vuksan V., Rao A.V., Thompson L.U., and Josse R.G. "Low Glycemic Index: Lente Carbohydrates and Physiological Effects of Altered Food Frequency." *American Journal of Clinical Nutrition*, 1994, 59:706S–709S.

Jenkins D.J.A., Wolever T.M.S., Vuksan V., Brighenti F., Cunnane S.C., Rao A.V., Jenkins A.L., Buckley G., Patten R., Singer W., Corey P., Josse R.G. "Nibbling versus Gorging: Metabolic Advantages of Increased Meal Frequency." *New England Journal of Medicine*, 1989; 321:929–934.

Maintain consistency to produce changes in taste preferences:

Mattes R.D. "Fat Preference and Adherence to a Reduced-fat Diet." *American Journal of Clinical Nutrition*, 1993; 57:373–381.

Van Horn L.V., Dolecek T.A., Grandits G.A., Skweres. "Adherence to Dietary Recommendations in the Special Intervention Group in the Multiple Risk Factor Intervention Trial." *American Journal of Clinical Nutrition* 1997; 65(suppl): 289S–304S.

Taste can change, depending on what you are used to eating:

Epstein L.H., Valoski A., Wing R.R., Perkins K.A., Fernstrom M., Marks B., and McCurley J. "Perception of Eating and Exercise in Children as a Function of Child and Parent Weight Status." *Appetite*, 1989; 12:105–118.

Mattes R.D. "Fat Preference and Adherence to a Reduced-fat Diet." *American Journal of Clinical Nutrition*, 1993; 57:373–381.

Urban N., White E., Anderson G.L., Curry S., and Kristal A.R. "Correlates of Maintenance of a Low-fat Diet among women in the Women's Health Trial." *Preventive Medicine*, 1992; 21(3):279–91.

Chapter 8: Triggers and the Net

Pate R.R., Pratt M., Blair S.N., Haskell W.L., Macera C.A., Bouchard C., Buchner D., Ettinger W., Heath G.W., and King A.C., et al. "Physical Activity and Public Health: A Recommendation from the Centers for Disease Control and Prevention and the American College of Sports Medicine." *Journal of the American Medical Association*, 1995; 273:402–7.

Walking is an aerobic exercise, which can strengthen heart, lungs, muscles, bones:

Blair S.N., Kohl H.W., Gordon N.F., and Paffenbarger R.S., Jr. "How Much Physical Activity Is Good for Health?" *Annual Review of Public Health*, 1992, 13:99–126.

Elward K. and Larson E.B. "Benefits of Exercise for Older Adults: A Review of Existing Evidence and Current Recommendations for the General Population." *Clinics in Geriatric Medicine*, 1992 February, 8(1):35–50.

Evans W.J. "Exercise, Nutrition, and Aging." *Clinics in Geriatric Medicine*, 1995 November, 11(4):725–34.

Running and brisk walking can raise HDL levels, which can reduce risk of heart disease and stroke:

Williams P.T. "High-density Lipoprotein Cholesterol and Other Risk Factors for Coronary Heart Disease in Female Runners." [see comments] *New England Journal of Medicine*, 1996 May 16, 334(20):1298–303.

Moderate exercise performed frequently boosts immune system and protects against cancer:

Elward K. and Larson E.B. "Benefits of Exercise for Older Adults: A Review of Existing Evidence and Current Recommendations for the General Population." *Clinics in Geriatric Medicine*, 1992 February, 8(1):35–50.

Exercise increases body's demand for fuel and burns calories stored as fat, thereby reducing body fatness and excess weight:

Ready A.E., Naimark B., Ducas J., Sawatzky J.V., Boreskie S.L., Drinkwater D.T., and Oosterveen S. "Influence of Walking Volume on Health Benefits in Women Post-menopause." *Medicine and Science in Sports and Exercise*, 1996 September, 28(9):1097–105.

Adoption of exercise elevates mood and relieves depression:

Ossip-Klein D.J., Doyne E.J., Bowman E.D., Osborn K.M., McDougall-Wilson I.B., and Neimeyer R.A. "Effects of Running or Weight Lifting on Self-concept in Clinically Depressed Women." *Journal of Consulting and Clinical Psychology*, 57, 158–161.

Pronk N.P., Crouse S.F., and Rohack J.J. "Maximal Exercise and Acute Mood Response in Women." *Physiology and Behavior*, 1995 January, 57(1):1–4.

Yeung R.R. "The Acute Effects of Exercise on Mood State." *Journal of Psychosomatic Research*, 1996 February, 40(2):123–41.

Having exercise facilities nearby facilitates attendance:

Sallis J.F., Hovell M.F., Hofstetter C.R., Elder J.P., Hackley M., Caspersen C.J., and Powell K.E. "Distance Between Homes and Exercise Facilities Related to Frequency of Exercise among San Diego Residents." *Public Health Reports*, 1990 March–April, 105(2):179–85.

Mornings are best time to exercise; those who exercise in morning have better adherence:

Atkinson G. and Reilly T. "Effects of Age and Time of Day on Preferred Work Rates during Prolonged Exercise." *Chronobiology International*, 1995 April, 12(2): 121–34.

Especially when it gets cold in the Fall, and less so during winter is time when people eat heavier meals:

de Castro J.M. "Seasonal Rhythms of Human Nutrient Intake and Meal Pattern." *Physiology and Behavior*, 1991 July, 50(1):243–8.

Seligson F.H., Krummel D.A., and Apgar J.L. "Patterns of chocolate consumption." *American Journal of Clinical Nutrition*, 1994 December, 60(6 Suppl): 1060S–1064S.

Soup provides bulk without too many calories and is satisfying:

Foreyt J.P., Reeves R.S., Darnell L.S., Wohlleb J.C., and Gotto A.M. "Soup Consumption as a Behavioral Weight Loss Strategy." *Journal of the American Dietetic Association*, 1986 April, 86(4):524–6.

Going to high-risk situation hungry conduces to relapse more than going full:

Shopping while hungry conduces to buying less healthful foods:

Beneke W.M. and Davis C.H. "Relationship of Hunger: Use of a Shopping List and Obesity to Food Purchases." *International Journal of Obesity*, 1985, 9(6):391–9.

Tom G. "Effect of Deprivation on the Grocery Shopping Behavior of Obese and Nonobese Consumers." *International Journal of Obesity*, 1983, 7(4):307–11.

Thorogood M., Mann J., Appleby P., and McPherson K. "Risk of Death from Cancer and Ischemic Heart Disease in Meat and Non-meat Eaters." *British Medical Journal*, 1994; 308:1667–1671.

Weight lifting is good for even ninety year olds:

Fiatarone M.A., O'Neill E.F., Ryan N.D., Clements K.M., Solares G.R., Nelson M.E., Roberts S.B., Kehayias J.J., Lipsitz L.A., and Evans W.J. "Exercise Training and Nutritional Supplementation for Physical Frailty in Very Elderly People." *New England Journal of Medicine*, 1994 June 23, 330(25):1769–75.

Bigger muscles from resistance training can help regulate blood glucose levels, which allows more fat-burning:

Kirwan J.P., Kohrt W.M., Wojta D.M., Bourey R.E., and Holloszy J.O. "Endurance Exercise Training Reduces Glucose-stimulated Insulin Levels in 60- to 70-year-old Men and Women." *Journal of Gerontology*, 1993 May, 48(3):M84–90.

Ryan A.S., Pratley R.E., Goldberg A.P., and Elahi D. "Resistive Training Increases Insulin Action in Postmenopausal Women." *Journals of Gerontology. Series A, Biological Sciences and Medical Sciences*, 1996 September, 51(5):M199–205.

Tarahumara Indians have low rates of heart disease. They have low cholesterol levels and they are lean:

McMurry M.P., Connor W.E., and Cerqueira M.T. "Dietary Cholesterol and the Plasma Lipids and Lipoproteins in the Tarahumara Indians: A People Habituated to a Low-cholesterol Diet after Weaning." *American Journal of Clinical Nutrition*, 1982 April, 35(4):741–4.

Connors got Tarahumara Indians to eat western diet, with predictably negative results for lipids:

McMurray M.P., Connor W.E., Lin D.S., Cerqueira M.T., and Connor S.L. "The Absorption of Cholesterol and the Sterol Balance in the Tarahumara Indians of Mexico Fed Cholesterol-free and High-cholesterol Diets." *American Journal of Clinical Nutrition*, 1985 June, 41(6):1289–98.

Fat instinct can be triggered by emotional or psychological threat:

Mitchell S.L. and Epstein L.H. "Changes in Taste and Satiety in Dietary-restrained Women Following Stress. *Physiology and Behavior*, 1996 August, 60(2):495–9.

It helps, in combating the fat instinct, to identify high-risk situations and to prepare for them:

Lorenz R.A., Bubb J., Davis D., Jacobson A., Jannasch K., Kramer J., Lipps J., and Schlundt D. "Changing Behavior: Practical Lessons from the Diabetes Control and Complications Trial." *Diabetes Care*, 1996 June, 19(6):648–52.

Appendix: Special Recommendations for People Suffering from Atherosclerosis, High Blood Pressure and Those Who Feel That They Are Losing Too Much Weight on the Pritikin Program

Plaques are the underlying cause of most heart attacks and strokes:

Braunwald, E., ed. *Heart Disease: A Textbook of Cardiovascular Medicine* 4th edition. Philadelphia: W.B. Saunders, 1992.

Atherosclerosis strikes when blood cholesterol levels become excessive:

Roberts W.C. "Preventing and Arresting Coronary Atherosclerosis." *American Heart Journal*, 1995 September, 130(3 Pt 1):580–600.

Scientists now believe that more immediate protection is afforded by eating a healthy diet than was presumed by Ornish when he tested a variant of the Pritikin dietary plan:

Treasure C.B., Klein J.L., Weintraub W.S., Talley J.D., Stillabower M.E., Kosinski A.S., Zhang J., Boccuzzi S.J., Cedarholm J.C., and Alexander R.W. "Beneficial Effects of Cholesterol-lowering Therapy on the Coronary Endothelium in Patients with Coronary Artery Disease." [see comments] *New England Journal of Medicine*, 1995 February 23, 332(8):481–7.

Plaques can be stabilized in a matter of weeks when shifting to a healthier diet and doing physical activity:

"Review of the Major Intervention Trials of Lowering Coronary Artery Disease Risk through Cholesterol Reduction." *American Journal of Cardiology*, 1996 September 26, 78(6A):13–9.

Factor VII:

Miller G.J. "Lipoproteins and the Haemostatic System in Atherothrombotic Disorders." *Baillieres Clinical Haematology*, 1994 September, 7(3):713–32.

Rosito G.B. and Tofler G.H. "Hemostatic Factors as Triggers of Cardiovascular Events." *Cardiology Clinics*, 1996 May, 14(2):239–50.

Soluble fibers have been shown to bind with fat and cholesterol in the intestinal tract and eliminate it from the body, thereby lowering overall blood cholesterol:

Kishimoto Y., Wakabayashi S., and Takeda H. "Hypocholesterolemic Effect of Dietary Fiber: Relation to Intestinal Fermentation and Bile Acid Excretion." *Journal of Nutritional Science and Vitaminology*, 1995 February, 41(1):151–61.

Beans and soybean products have been especially potent at lowering blood cholesterol because of soluble fibers, as well as high amount of vegetable protein. Vegetable protein independently lowers blood cholesterol:

Anderson J.W., Johnstone B.M., and Cook-Newell M.E. "Meta-analysis of the Effects of Soy Protein Intake on Serum Lipids." [see comments] *New England Journal of Medicine*, 1995 August 3, 333(5):276–82.

Animal protein increases blood cholesterol:

Ishinaga M., Hamada M., Ohnaka K., Fukunaga K., and Minato Y. "Effects of Casein and Soy Protein on Accumulation of Cholesterol and Dolichol in Rat Liver." *Proceedings of the Society for Experimental Biology and Medicine*, 1993 May,

Meal frequency influences blood cholesterol:

Jenkins D.J., Jenkins A.L., Wolever T.M., Vuksan V., Rao A.V., Thompson L.U., and Josse R.G. "Low Glycemic Index: Lente Carbohydrates and Physiological Effects of Altered Food Frequency." *American Journal of Clinical Nutrition*, 1994 March, 59(3 Suppl):706S–709S.

Exercise lowers triglycerides and blood pressure:

Williams P. T. "Relationship of Distance Run per Week to Coronary Heart Disease Risk Factors in 8,283 Male Runners." *The National Runners' Health Study.* [see comments] *Archives of Internal Medicine*, 1997 January 27, 157(2):191–8.

Exercise tends to raise HDL:

Williams P.T. "High-density Lipoprotein Cholesterol and Other Risk Factors for Coronary Heart Disease in Female Runners." *New England Journal of Medicine*, 1996; 334:1298–1303.

Aspirin may help to prevent blood clots:

"Aspirin to Prevent Heart Attack or Stroke." *Drug and Therapeutics Bulletin,* 1994 January 20, 32(1):1–3.

Pritikin experience helps blood lipids:

Barnard R.J. "Effects of Life-style Modification on Serum Lipids." *Archives of Internal Medicine,* 1991; 151:1389–1394.

Pritikin has good track record for restoring diabetics to better functioning:

Barnard R.J., Jung T., and Inkeles S.B. "Diet and Exercise in the Treatment of NIDDM." *Diabetes Care,* 1994; 17:1469–1472.

Barnard R.J., Massey M.R., Cherny S., O'Brien L.T., and Pritikin N. "Long-term Use of a High-complex-carbohydrate, High-fiber, Low-fat diet, and Exercise in the Treatment of NIDDM Patients." *Diabetes Care,* 1983 May–June, 6(3):268–73.

Sodium chloride is important contributor to hypertension:

Dyer A.R., Elliott P., and Shipley M. for the InterSalt Cooperative Research Group. "Urinary Electrolyte Excretion in 24 Hours and Blood Pressure in the INTER-SALT Study II. Estimates of Electrolyte-blood Pressure Associations Corrected for Regression Dilution Bias." *American Journal of Epidemiology,* 1994; 139: 940–951.

Houston M.C. "Sodium and Hypertension." *Archives of Internal Medicine,* 1986; 146:179–185.

Minimum and maximum recommended intakes of sodium:

Excess salt intake contributes to calcium excretion, which can be expected to produce osteoporosis:

National Research Council. *Recommended Dietary Allowances.* Washington, D.C.: National Academy Press, 1989.

O'Brien K.O., Abrams S.A., Stuff J.E., Liang L.K., and Welch T.R. "Variables Related to Urinary Calcium Excretion in Young Girls." *Journal of Pediatric Gastroenterology and Nutrition,* 1996 July, 23(1):8–12.

Excess salt intake produces kidney stones:

Massey L.K. and Whiting S.J. "Dietary Salt, Urinary Calcium, and Kidney Stone Risk." *Nutrition Reviews,* 1995 May, 53(5):131–9.

High fat diets contribute to high blood pressure:

Rantala M., Savolainen M.J., Kervinen K., and Kesaniemi Y.A. "Apolipoprotein E Phenotype and Diet-induced Alteration in Blood Pressure." *American Journal of Clinical Nutrition,* 1997 February, 65(2):543–50.

Obesity contributes to high blood pressure:

Ascherio A., Hennekens C., Willett W.C., Sacks F., Rosner B., Manson J., Witteman J., and Stampfer M.J. "Prospective Study of Nutritional Factors, Blood Pressure, and Hypertension among U.S. Women." *Hypertension*, 1996 May, 27(5): 1065–72.

"Effects of weight loss and sodium reduction intervention on blood pressure and hypertension incidence in overweight people with high-normal blood pressure. The Trials of Hypertension Prevention, phase II. The Trials of Hypertension Prevention Collaborative Research Group." [see comments] *Archives of Internal Medicine*, 1997 March 24, 157(6):657–67.

Kannel W.B. "Blood Pressure as a Cardiovascular Risk Factor: Prevention and Treatment." [see comments] *JAMA*, 1996 May 22–29, 275(20):1571–6.

Srinivasan S.R., Bao W., Wattigney W.A., and Berenson G.S. "Adolescent Overweight Is Associated with Adult Overweight and Related Multiple Cardiovascular Risk Factors: The Bogalusa Heart Study." *Metabolism: Clinical and Experimental*, 1996 February, 45(2):235–40.

Too much alcohol contributes to high blood pressure:

Ascherio A., Hennekens C., Willett W.C., Sacks F., Rosner B., Manson J., Witteman J., and Stampfer M.J. "Prospective Study of Nutritional Factors, Blood Pressure, and Hypertension among U.S. Women." *Hypertension*, 1996 May, 27(5): 1065–72.

Krogh V., Trevisan M., Jossa F., Farinaro E., Panico S., Mancini M., Menotti A., and Ricci G. "Alcohol and Blood Pressure: The Effects of Age." Findings from the Italian Nine Communities Study. The Research Group ATS-RF2 of the Italian National Research Council. *Annals of Epidemiology*, 1993 May, 3(3):245–9.

Wakabayashi K., Nakamura K., Kono S., Shinchi K., and Imanishi K. "Alcohol Consumption and Blood Pressure: An Extended Study of Self-defence Officials in Japan." *International Journal of Epidemiology*, 1994 April, 23(2):307–11.

Diets low in calcium contribute to high blood pressure:

Appel L.J., Moore T.J., Obarzanek E., Vollmer W.M., Svetkey L.P., Sacks F.M., Bray G.A., Vogt T.M., Cutler J.A., and Windhauser M.M., et al. "A Clinical Trial of the Effects of Dietary Patterns on Blood Pressure." DASH Collaborative Research Group. *New England Journal of Medicine*, 1997 April 17, 336(16): 1117–24.

McCarron D.A. "Role of Adequate Dietary Calcium Intake in the Prevention and Management of Salt-sensitive Hypertension." *American Journal of Clinical Nutrition*, 1997 February, 65(2 Suppl):712S–716S.

Diets low in potassium contribute to high blood pressure:

Tobian L. "Dietary Sodium Chloride and Potassium Have Effects on the Pathophysiology of Hypertension in Humans and Animals." *American Journal of Clinical Nutrition*, 1997 February, 65(2 Suppl):606S–611S.

Diets low in magnesium contribute to high blood pressure:

McCarron D.A. "Role of Adequate Dietary Calcium Intake in the Prevention and Management of Salt-sensitive Hypertension." *American Journal of Clinical Nutrition*, 1997 February, 65(2 Suppl):712S–716S.

Most important factor besides diet for affecting high blood pressure is exercise:

Beilin L., Burke V., and Milligan R. "Strategies for Prevention of Adult Hypertension and Cardiovascular Risk Behaviour in Childhood: An Australian Perspective." *Journal of Human Hypertension*, 1996 February, 10 Suppl 1:S51–4.

Pritikin has been successful in reducing blood pressure and getting people off of blood pressure medication:

Barnard R.J., Ugianskis E.J., Martin D.A., and Inkeles S.B. "Role of Diet and Exercise in the Management of Hyperinsulinemia and Associated Atherosclerotic Risk Factors." *American Journal of Cardiology*, 1992 February 15, 69(5):440–4.

Research has shown that men and women who are consistently through the lifespan below the average in weight live longer:

Manson, J.E., Stampfer, M.J., Hennekens, C.H., and Willet, W.C. "Body weight and longevity." *Journal of the American Medical Association*, 1987; 257, 353–358.
Manson J.E., Willett W.C., Stampfer M.J., Colditz G.A., Hunter D.J., Hankinson S.E., Hennekens C.H., and Speizer F.E. "Body Weight and Mortality among Women." *The New England Journal of Medicine*, 1995; 333:677–685.

Weight training can offset tendency to lose muscle during weight loss:

Zachwieja J.J. "Exercise as Treatment for Obesity." *Endocrinology and Metabolism Clinics of North America*, 1996 December, 25(4):965–88.

Intake of more more nuts may protect against heart attack and lower cholesterol level:

Dreher M.L., Maher C.V., and Kearney P. "The Traditional and Emerging Role of Nuts in Healthful Diets." *Nutrition Reviews*, 1996 August, 54(8):241–5.

Force-feeding carbs to gain weight raises triglycerides:

Schaefer E.J., Lichtenstein A.H., Lamon-Fava S., McNamara J.R., Schaefer M.M., Rasmussen H., and Ordovas J.M. "Body Weight and Low-density Lipoprotein Cholesterol Changes after Consumption of a Low-fat Ad Libitum Diet." [see comments] JAMA, 1995 November 8, 274(18):1450–5.

INDEX